UNDERSTANDING

Arthritis

The Silent Menace Within

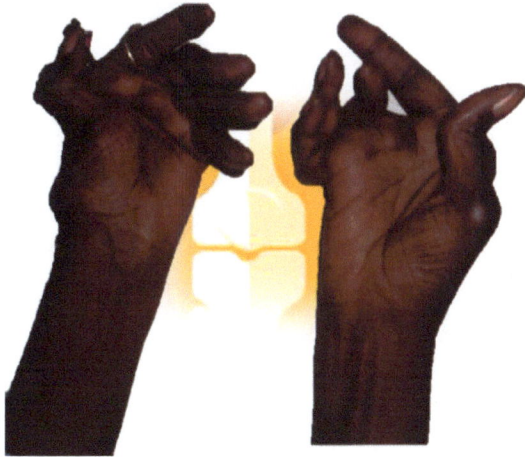

UNDERSTANDING

Arthritis

The Silent Menace Within

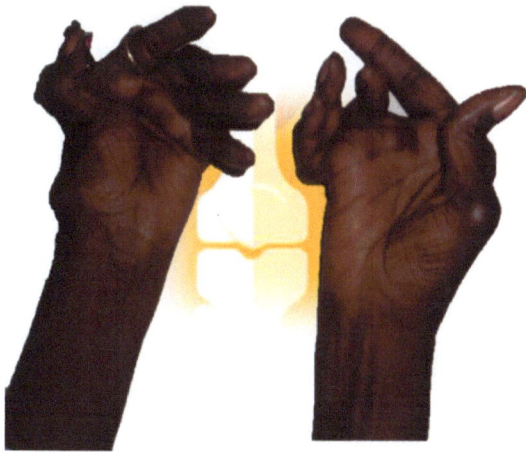

Dr. Omondi Oyoo
FACR; FRCP (Edin); MMed; MB Ch B

Published by Sahel Publishing Association
P.O. Box 18007—00100
Nairobi, Kenya
Tel: +011-254-715-596-106
www.sahelpublishing.net
Narrated by Sam Okello

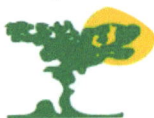

A Sahel Book
Editor: Sam Okello
Interior design: Hellen Wahonya Okello
Cover design: Peter Omamo
Images: Dr. Omondi Oyoo and Google Images
Author contact: Dr. Omondi Oyoo
Tel: +254-727-935706
Printed in India

This book is deservedly dedicated to my wife and best friend, Eunice, and to our daughters Barbara, Sheila and Ivy, all who made it possible for me to find time to write this book; and to my mom, Monica, Auntie Appelles and Grandmother Abisage (now deceased): they have all endured the pain of living with knee joint arthritis; and to all patients with arthritis who are going through great suffering and have been devastated by the pain that arthritis brings— you have not suffered your affliction and pain in vain; one glad morning the Lord will declare all pain OVER!

Foreword

If there were to be any single terms describing the book you are holding in your hands, they would easily include: *Terrific, Fantastic, Readable, Timely, Authoritative, Friendly and Frank*!

And whereas self-help books abound in many fields today (including from redoubtable quacks), it is not always the case that you will find one book that answers your needs so personally and so compassionately; more so in a Kenyan, African context. The situation is certainly much dire in the field of Medicine where most of us routinely resign our fate to the wisdom of doctors, (that is assuming you are lucky enough to access one in good time).

Therefore, *getting educated* about an ailment-as my friend Dr. Oyoo counsels here—certainly forestalls the full and painful impact of the many mysterious maladies that have become the bane of humankind today.

Arthritis—or simply—the bone and joint disease—in my layman's reading—is one such malady. And behold; so many than YOU imagine, are quietly suffering, completely unable to comprehend what might have happened to their once strong and energetic limbs. This disease is often debilitating in its onset with acute, inexplicable pain. We are told it has the potential to completely paralyze; maim; kill, or just completely remove its victim from any gainful or joyous engagement in life.

The one myth that Dr. Oyoo disabuses us of quite early in the book, is also the idea that Arthritis is a disease for the aged; oh not at all! It can actually afflict children as young as seven years and it is far more widespread than we think. Its many manifestations include, not just the much better— known Gout (that so painfully attacks the many connoisseurs of Kenya's *nyama choma* (roast meat) culture and alcohol; but there are others: rheumatoid; LUPUS (the type that for some reason, prefers to mainly attack females); the reactive type as well as osteoarthritis. Invariably, in all these painful conditions could also be the consequence of our own lifestyles and particularly, that common middle class refusal to see value in exercise, or even live by healthier diets as ordered by the doctor.

In this book, Dr. Oyoo—in a truly philanthropic fashion—has offered an eye opening Patient Education remedy that must be a major precursor to the urgent need for more widespread Public Health Education programs covering the whole array of ailments. Perhaps in retrospect, one can say that the presumption that it was only HIV/AIDS that needed this kind of attention was erroneous; particularly in the wake of such pervasive ignorance around so many other 'silent menaces' and killers such as high blood pressure; cancer, Arthritis...that lot!

I want to commend Dr. Omondi Oyoo for doing a really brilliant job in demystifying the *mumbo-jumbo* we often associate with Medicine. The descriptions of various Arthritic conditions with such convincing reliance on patient case studies has been so eloquently told with appropriate pictorial illustration; diagnosis procedures and available treatment options. But above all, it rings with palpable authority, clearly emanating from the pen of a professional who has prioritized and specialized in this area of practice over so many years. In a sense, Dr. Oyoo has also contributed to the growth of Kenyan Literature; specifically the unique genre of Medical Narratives; up to now dominated by the one Dr. Yusuf Kodavwala Dawood and made so popular through 'Surgeons Diary' run in the Kenyan popular press.

This is a patient-centered mandatory reading that I must readily recommend to every man and woman: it will enable YOU, to take charge of your life in good time to live a long productive life while also avoiding those crippling and often-runaway medical bills.

Dr. George Odera Outa (LLB Hons (Lon); BA; MA (Nrb); PhD (Wits).
Lecturer and Independent Consultant:
University of Nairobi, College of Humanities and Social Sciences.

ACKNOWLEDGEMENT

I want to thank each of the people I've mentioned in this page for the help they extended my way in my journey to becoming the doctor I am today and in the journey to writing this book:

Editors:
Sam Okello
Hellen Wahonya Okello
Philip Ojwang

Family:
Eunice Mildred Akinyi Omondi
Barbara Awuor Omondi
Sheila Ajwang Omondi
Ivy Achieng Oyoo

Mentors:
Yair Molad(Israel), Luis Espinoza(Louisiana, USA)
Girish Mody(South Africa), Asgar Ali Kalla (South Africa)
Bill Lore (Kenya), Joseph Amolo Aluoch (Kenya)
Elijah Ogola (Kenya)

Great Teacher and Mentor:
Arthur Othieno Obel

Nairobi Arthritis Clinic Staff:
Susan Othieno
Winifred Musyoka

Publisher:
Sahel Publishing Association

Table of Contents

Foreword.. ix

Acknowledgement... xiii

Introduction.. 17

Chapter One
Arthritis In Children.. 21

Chapter Two
Rheumatoid Arthritis....................................... 35

Chapter Three
Reactive Arthritis.. 46

Chapter Four
Osteoarthritis.. 57

Chapter Five
Gout... 76

Chapter Six
Lupus (Systematic Erythematous)........................... 89

Chapter Seven
Patient Education... 97

Introduction

Mary came to my office, along 5th Ngong Avenue, Nairobi, late in the evening in a lot of pain. She had just been rushed in for an appointment made the day before through my secretary. In deep distress, Mary had traveled from Kisii, some three hundred kilometers, in a speeding bus and was now near tears with excruciating pain. I advised the secretary to skip the preliminaries and let the lady in. As soon as she got into the examination room and saw a chair, she dived into it and grimaced in a manner I had never seen any other patient do before.

Over the years, I have treated thousands of arthritics and come to the conclusion that many patients suffering this malady lack the barest knowledge to deal with it or even manage it. Many people don't know that there are preventive measures one can take to either slow down its onset or keep its symptoms at bay altogether.

Having examined Mary that evening, and concerned that she had lived with this silent, excruciating pain without knowing what was eating her bones, as she put it, I decided the time had come to write a book on this disease. I wanted to develop a simple book that anybody could read and have a basic understanding of the cause, effects, types and other matters related to this disease. Does that mean there is no literature on it? Not at all; what it means is that the books and other available literature written on arthritis are elitist and are not designed to impart knowledge to Wanjiku (common man); they are designed to refresh the memory of the likes of Dr. Oyoo and other medical practitioners.

And so this book is written primarily for the many people out there who wallow in chronic or long-term pain. Many people with chronic diseases such as arthritis live with pain for years. Diseases of the nerves (trigeminal neuralgia, for example), shingles and nerve damage from injury or surgery can also be the cause of pain. Some people learn to cope with the help of drugs, physical treatments and other techniques; others find the pain more difficult to deal with and suffer in prolonged silence just like Mary did. The danger is that the pain may become a dominating and negative force in the life of the victim.

The good news for Mary and others in her situation is that increasingly there are new approaches to the management of arthritic pain and other pains in general. These can be helpful even if the victim is already coping well. One of the keys to handling pain is understanding it. It's thus important to understand the following:

- The available treatments
- What the treatments entail
- Why these treatments are helpful

On the other end of the (pain) spectrum, it is also crucial to understand:

- The pain itself
- Causes of the pain
- The different characteristics of the pain

Later in the book we will discuss pain briefly and tie it in with the different ways arthritis manifests in us today. In the case of Mary, her pain was so bad that I had to begin by administering a painkiller before engaging her in any manner. It is crucial that part of understanding this illness include an ability to detect its manifestations and a knowledge of when to seek help. Waiting too long to deal with it, as Mary did, can lead to the kind of pricking pain she experienced and even reduce the chances of successful treatment.

I do not guarantee whoever reads this book a place in the kingdom of health with regard to arthritis, but I can guarantee that whoever equips him/herself with the knowledge set in here will identify and deal with this illness as soon as the symptoms show. This knowledge may be the difference between a deeply cantankerous boss or husband and a joyous, achieving one. The time to act to take control of your total life is now, not when you turn sixty five as some folk think. Remember—life begins at sixty these days!

Dr. Omondi Oyoo, Arthritis Clinic Nairobi

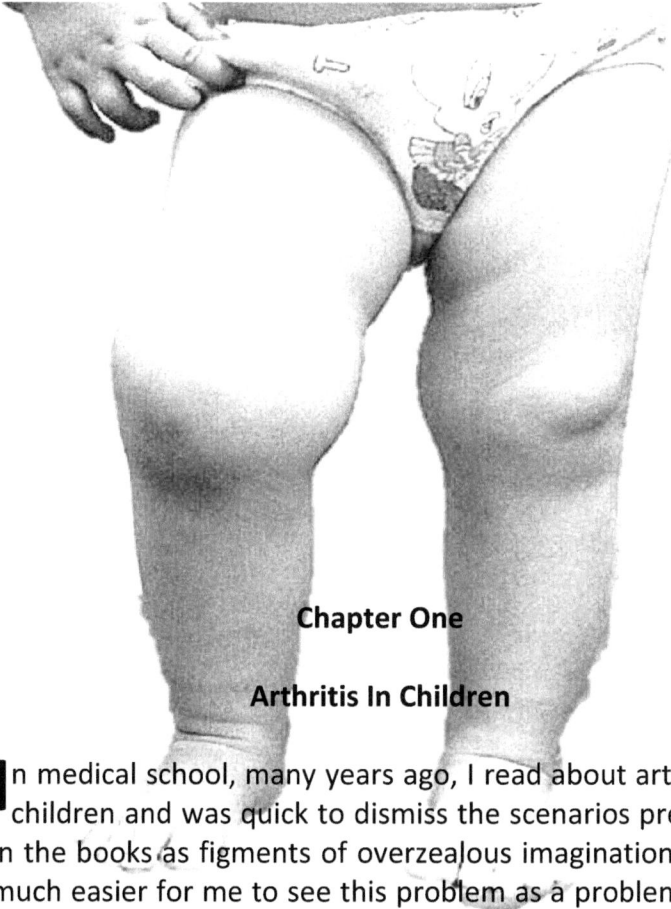

Chapter One

Arthritis In Children

In medical school, many years ago, I read about arthritis in children and was quick to dismiss the scenarios presented in the books as figments of overzealous imagination. It was much easier for me to see this problem as a problem of the aged, those whose tendons and ligaments had worn off due to the rubbing and grinding motions of the passage of time. Since that early encounter with the prospect of child arthritis, I have lived to see children afflicted.

I recall the evening I was in the office when a father and mother walked in and asked to see me. Looking at them, I thought one of them would tell me about their trouble with arthritis, but it didn't work that way. Within minutes of sitting across the desk from me, the mother breathlessly narrated how her daughter—a nine-year-old girl—had been going through trouble with what had since presented symptoms of arthritis.

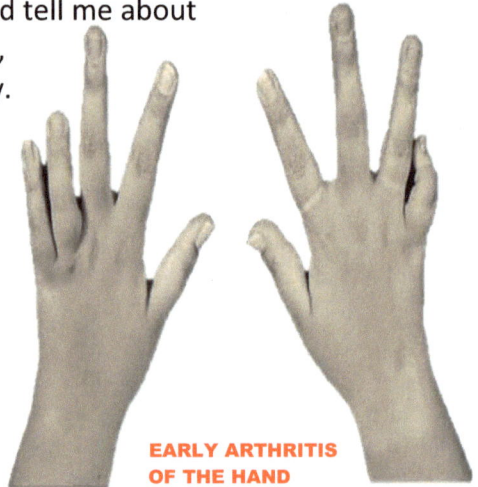

EARLY ARTHRITIS OF THE HAND

"How long has this been going on?" I asked the couple.

"Almost a year now," the mother said.

"And in all that time she hasn't received medical attention?"

The father said, "Doctor Oyoo, Nina has been seen by other doctors. The problem is—she is not getting any better; she is getting worse. This condition is beginning to affect her school work as well. We are here because we were referred by a friend. Our girl needs help." He bit his lip. "We can't go on like this!"

I can't say that Nina was the first child afflicted by arthritis that I ever met, but I must admit she was the most serious case. I was amazed by the depth of pain she was in and the inability of other doctors to treat her sooner. Looking at her, I thought of my own daughters and knew at once I had to act. Nina needed to be a normal child, to play like her friends and do the chores other kids did.

A Brief Background

Many people, even doctors, find it surprising to learn that children also suffer arthritis. When confronted with a case of arthritis in children, many physicians say there is nothing that can be done. Nothing can be farther from the truth; of course children can be helped and must be helped. Like adults, children have joints and those joints, for one reason or another, may be affected at an early age. Leaving them unattended as the children grow up is a disservice that we cannot let stand.

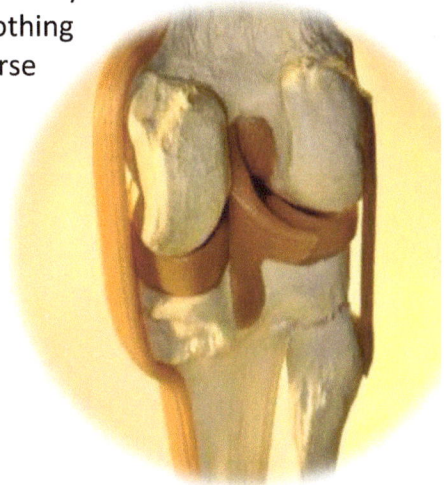

INSIDE THE KNEE JOINT

To have a clear understanding of this matter, let me begin by describing what a joint is. A joint is where two bones meet and move in relation to each other. Without a joint there could be no movement. The bone-ends are covered by cartilage and enclosed in a bag (capsule). These are in turn covered by a thin shiny membrane (synovium), which secretes the fluid that lubricates the joint (see image below).

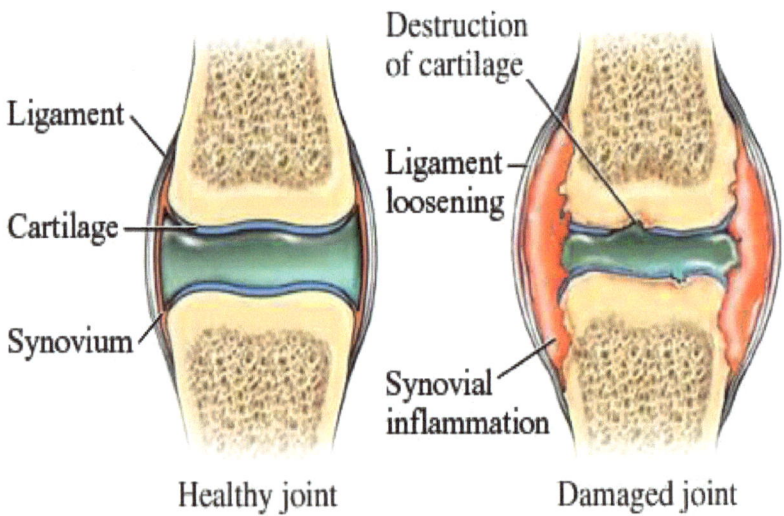

Healthy joint   Damaged joint

With the above discussion in mind, it shouldn't take a rocket scientist to figure out that either the cartilage or the membrane could be affected and thus cause trouble even for a child. In the event that it happens, that child needs immediate attention so that the problem does not snowball into something bigger and costlier to handle later.

So How Does Arthritis Affect Children?

Some of these medical terms have no easy translation and so allow me to be as basic as I can yet not lose sight of the description I must pass on. But before I do so, I should say from the onset that I wish to deal with the four prevalent forms of arthritis in children. I'll take them one by one.

(i) *Synovitis*

Arthritis (synovitis) is inflammation of the synovium lining the joint and—like a headache or a cough—it may be a symptom of many different diseases, some of which are acute, others chronic.

The cause of some form of arthritis (synovitis) in children is known. Injury and infection are among the commonest. That should come as no surprise because injury would result in painful swelling of the joint and is normally accompanied by bruising and abrasion of the skin, depending of course on the nature and severity of the accident.

FACIAL RASH IN JUVENILE ARTHRITIS

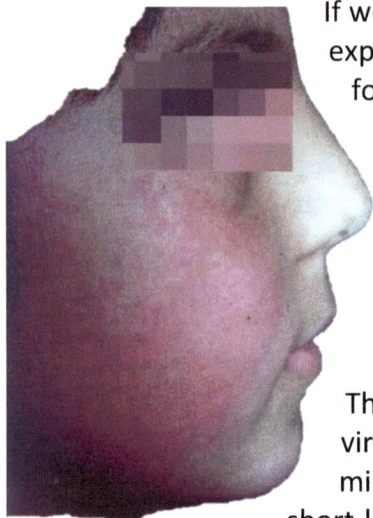

If we were to grade the level of pain a child experiences as a result of the different forms of arthritis, we would grade this form (synovitis) the highest. It is the kind that makes our children unable to be functional because of the pain emanating from dry joints.

(ii) *Viral Arthritis*

This is a form of arthritis caused by viruses. The good news is that it is usually mild and short-lived.

JUVENILE ARTHRITIS RASH

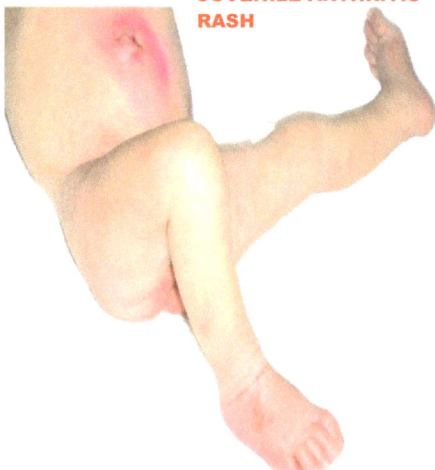

If a child were to be a victim of this form of arthritis, what the child needs is quick treatment and sufficient rest. That should take care of the problem at once.

(iii) *Bacterial Arthritis*

Bacterial arthritis is caused by bacteria. Let me be clear because this is serious. This form of arthritis is usually acute and may result in severe joint destruction. An early treatment with antibiotics is essential to prevent this.

Other Types Of Arthritis To Watch In Children

Rheumatic Fever

This type of arthritis is commonly associated with low socio-economic status and usually follows a throat infection. It may cause joint pains and swelling, but may also leave the heart valves damaged.

There are other types of arthritis whose causes no one knows, for example the one commonly known as Juvenile Chronic Arthritis (JCA). But like I said before, early treatment for a child attacked by any of these forms of arthritis is critical. This is because there are many cases that may be arrested or managed before they become a bigger and less easy to manage problem. Speed is of the essence here!

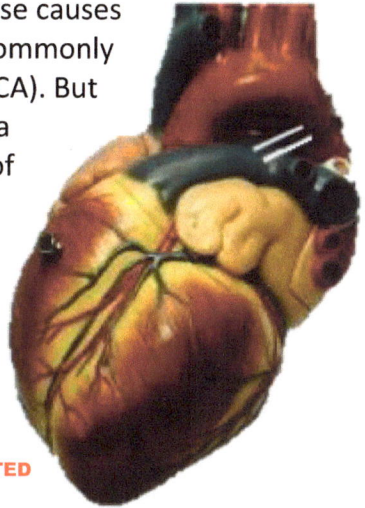

THE HEART; COMMONLY AFFECTED IN RHEUMATIC FEVER

Let's Talk About Symptoms In Children

An inflamed joint will produce the following symptoms:

SKIN REDNESS IN INFLAMMATION

- Pain
- Swelling
- Warmth
- Redness
- Stiffness
- Limitation of movement

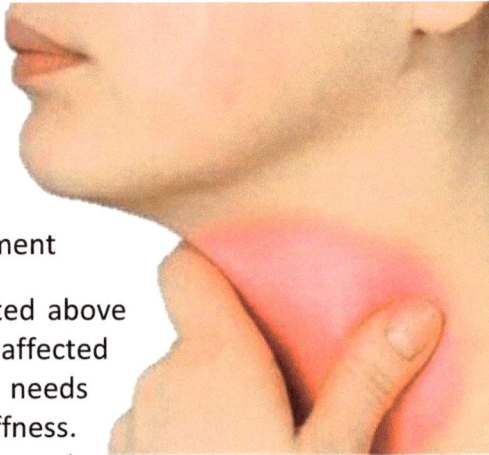

Most of the symptoms listed above are self-evident in a child affected by arthritis. The one that needs further mention is stiffness. Stiffness is most pronounced after periods of inactivity such as waking up in the morning, arising from a TV program or from a school desk at the end of a period. In such a case, one or many joints may be affected and this may cause reverberating pain.

Other noted symptoms in children include fever and skin rash. Swelling of the glands may also occur, especially in the neck and in the armpits. Children presenting with these symptoms are usually miserable, lethargic and may have poor appetite. They may complain of sore throat and show signs of tiring easily. Other organs such as the eyes, heart, liver, spleen and lungs may be involved.

It is easy to see that a child in this condition would be too miserable and may be unable to function normally. The word of the good doctor is this—get that child to his or her doctor at once for treatment. There can be no waiting!

Diagnosis

When Nina was brought to my office, I knew the range of tests I had to run. In the medical world, even if a patient comes to you and is so sure of the problem—and even the doctor is pretty certain the patient is right—tests should still be done to confirm those suspicions. And so when Nina was brought in, in spite of the fact that I was sure she was afflicted by one form of arthritis or another, I subjected her to tests to confirm the fears, then zeroed-in-on which type.

Let me paint a general picture of the process. When a patient walks in, the patient is examined fully. X-rays are done to check that the heart and lungs are healthy and to see if any bone or joint changes have occurred. Blood is taken to exclude anemia and to look for rheumatoid factor. This is an antibody against normal antibody proteins, which is present in some of the patients. This usually portends a more serious and longer lasting disease.

Tests are also done to exclude other causes of arthritis and connective tissue diseases. Some of the tests commonly done include antinuclear antibody.

Some tests, when done, indicate an inherited susceptibility to certain types of arthritis; for instance, HLA-B27, which predisposes to arthritis of the spine (poker back).

The eyes must be examined with a special instrument called a slit-lamp, and this is repeated every six months. Now, this is another point where I need to get shrill: Inflammation in the eye in a juvenile (child) arthritis situation may go undetected and this could cause irreversible blindness.

And finally, fluid may be taken from the joint through a biopsy or removal of a piece of tissue of the synovial lining affected in the place where precise diagnosis is rendered impossible due to one circumstance or another. In Nina's case, I had to subject her to the range of tests I've mentioned because of the severity of her situation. By the time I was done, it was clear what we needed to do.

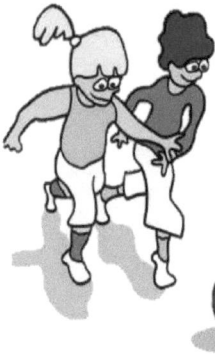

Treating Arthritis In Children

Let me begin by making a declarative statement that effective treatment for arthritis in children is available. This treatment is aimed at ushering the child to a "burnt-out" stage free of disability and deformity. To achieve this, a couple of factors must be put in place:

- Make an effort to relieve the pain and stiffness
- Encourage activity and maintain mobility

As I worked with Nina, I had to take into account the fact that each child is different, so I had to make a specific program of treatment, tailor-made for her. This individualized program would not be used on any other child or things would go wrong for that other child.

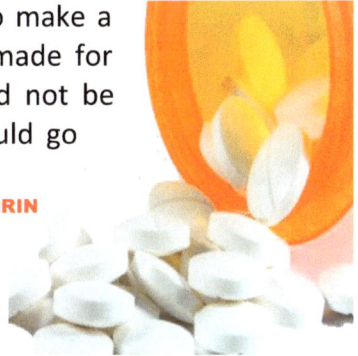

ASPIRIN

What Then Is Child-friendly Treatment?

1. *Aspirin and other non-steroidal anti-inflammatory drugs*

Firstly, inflammation may be suppressed by anti inflammatory drugs. The simplest is aspirin. There are many others. They are called Non-Steroidal Anti-Inflammatory Drugs (NSAIDs). These drugs have side effects so the choice of which one to use is governed by a child's response.

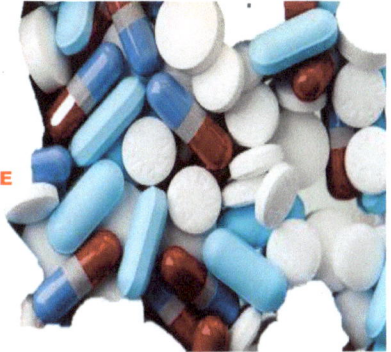

CORTISONE

2. *Cortisone (prednisone)* and disease modifying drugs

In a child with more serious disease, cortisone (prednisone) is used. The duration and dosage of this drug is kept low because there are more troublesome side effects. If these drugs don't work or provide incomplete resolution of joint inflammation, then slow-acting, disease modifying drugs like methotrexate may be used. These drugs, however, take a few months before any effect becomes noticeable. Their possible side effects necessitate regular follow up and frequent examination of the skin, blood and urine.

There are newer disease modifying drugs such as eternacept, which cause faster resolution of symptoms and could lead to remission of disease.

3. *Physical Therapy*

Physical therapy helps to preserve the range of motion of the joints, reduce joint injury, prevent the joints from becoming bent, and maintain muscle strength. Anti-inflammatory drug treatment should be regarded as a means to reducing pain and swelling so that physical therapy can be undertaken. Also helpful are splints and exercises in a heated pool (hydrotherapy).

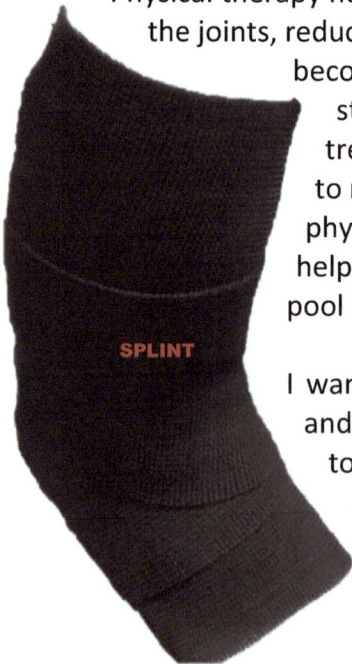

SPLINT

I want to conclude this chapter on children and arthritis by saying this—children need to be helped as soon as symptoms of the more problematic arthritis show. While a doctor is eventually the leader in a treatment situation, help must be coordinated at home, at school and all the places a child goes to. Any activity that causes further strain in a child diagnosed with any form of arthritis must be discouraged and minimized.

Now that I have dealt with arthritis in children, I feel free to handle this malady in adults. Because of the varied ways this illness presents in adults, I want to discuss the types first.

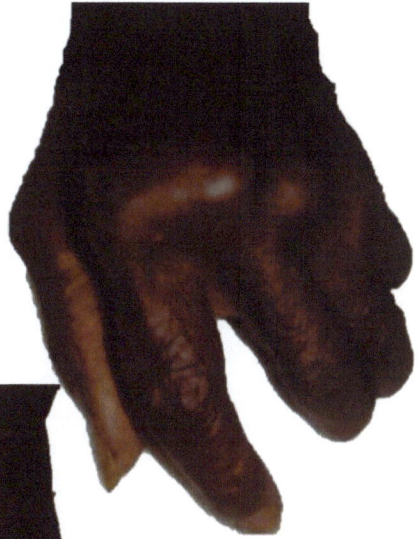

HAND DEFORMITY IN ARTHRITIS

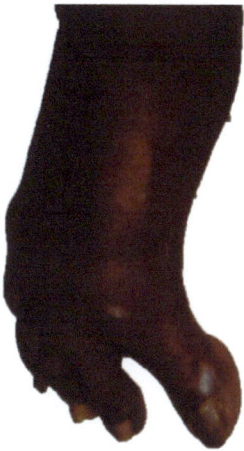

FEET DEFORMITY IN ARTHRITIS

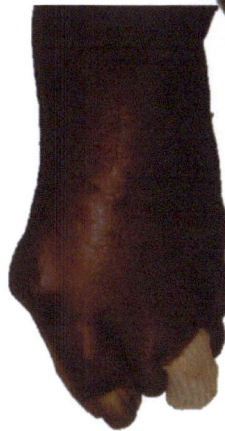

4. Patient Education

But before we go to types, let me say something about patient education. Patient education is critical in the management of arthritis, whether in children or in adults. Because the factors involved in educating patients are the same through the spectrum of age, I will discuss these factors together at the end of this book under the subtitle, Patient Education.

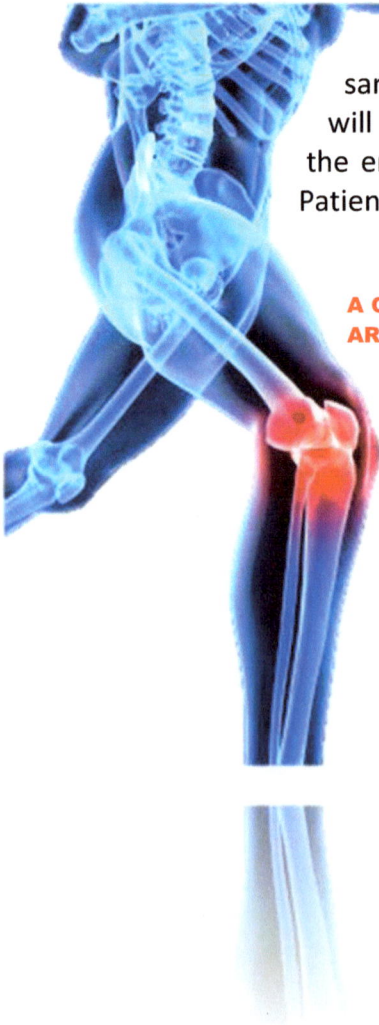

A CARICATURE OF AN ARTHRITIC PATIENT JOGGING

Chapter Two

Rheumatoid Arthritis

In chapter one, because we were dealing with children, we defined arthritis in pretty general terms, so before we delve deeper into what rheumatoid arthritis is, let me broaden the scope of things a bit. Arthritis, for the purposes of this new level of discussion, is a term that basically refers to diseases of the joints, mostly presenting as inflammations of the joints. Arthritis normally presents as pain, hotness, swelling, or loss of function of a joint. There are about 200 different types of this condition.

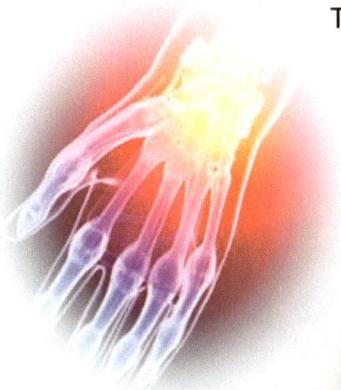

INFLAMMED FINGERS

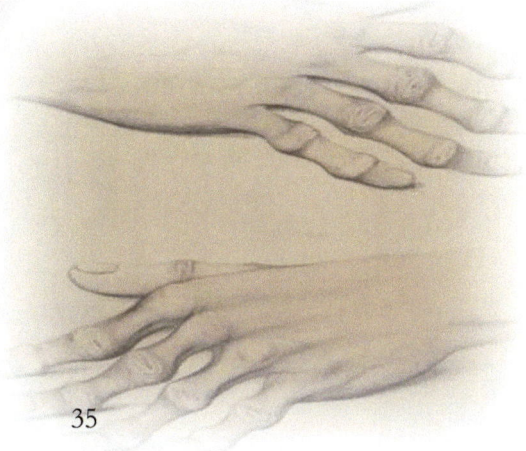

HAND ARTHRITIS

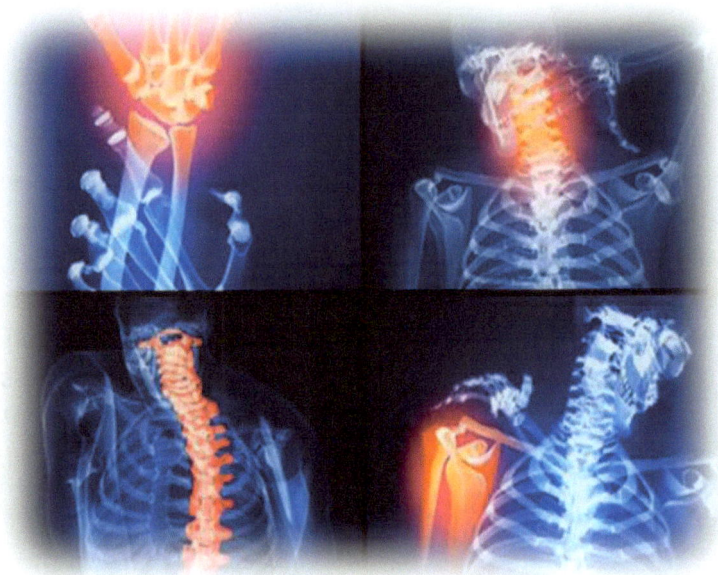

ARTHRITIS OF VARIOUS JOINTS

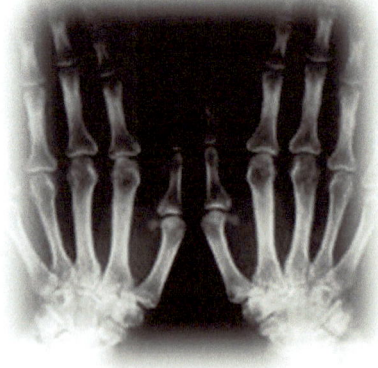

A joint is the meeting point of bones. Our joints enable us to perform many different functions in the body such as movement, eating, bending, squatting, standing, turning the neck and bending the back. The many joints in the body include:

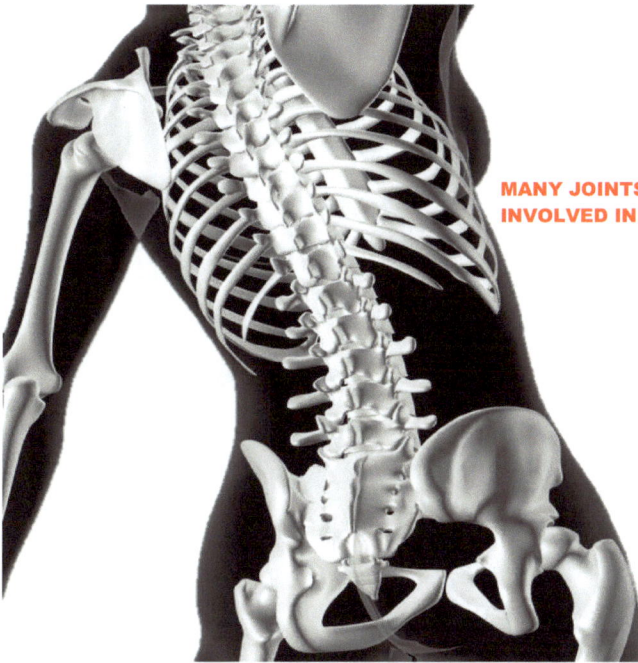

MANY JOINTS CAN BE INVOLVED IN ARTHRITIS

- Knee
- Elbow
- Shoulder
- Back etc

Though the bones articulate (turn) at the joints, they are held together by muscles, tendons, ligaments and capsules.

These are important in giving firmness to the joints and they also maintain the integrity of the joints by facilitating smooth movement of one bone over another. Without these tissues we would run the risk of tearing our joints any time we moved.

What Is Rheumatoid Arthritis?

RHEUMATOID HAND DEFORMITY

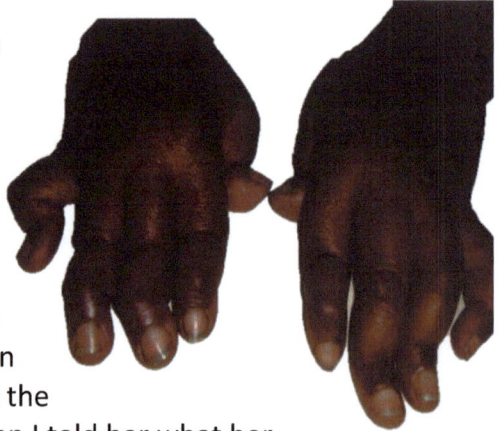

In this book's introduction, I told of a visit I had with Mary. The lady had just arrived in Nairobi from Kisii to get treatment from me. After a series of tests were conducted by my staff, I came to settle on rheumatoid arthritis as the culprit in her case. When I told her what her problem was, she promptly asked what rheumatoid arthritis was. She wanted a description. This is what I told Mary:

Rheumatoid arthritis is a chronic debilitating autoimmune disease in which the immune system attacks healthy tissue. More than twenty million folks worldwide are affected by it.

When in its element, it is a destructive type of arthritis that affects joints, muscles, tendons and other structures surrounding the joints. You can immediately see why it is one of the most painful and frustrating forms of this problem.

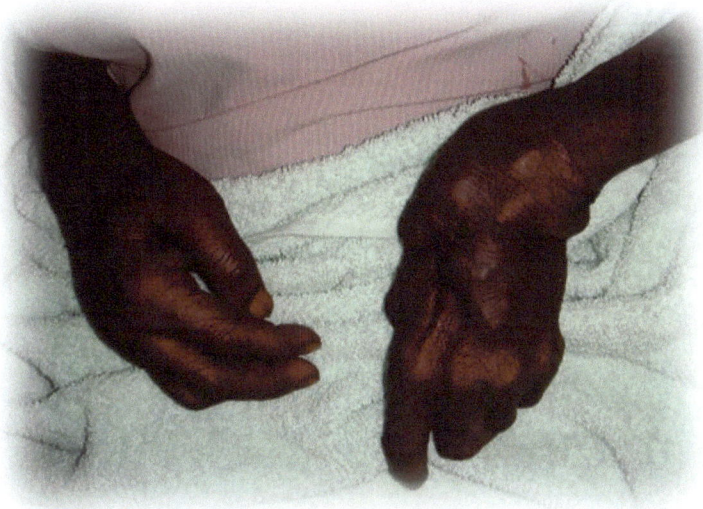

RHEUMATOID HAND

Being an autoimmune disease, it does something that should not happen in the body. It makes room for the white blood cells, which should protect the body, to start acting crazy and destroy the body instead. In other words, this is a situation where the soldiers (white blood cells) carry out a coup against the body. Why this happens nobody knows; all we know is that it does happen. Some researchers have suggested a possible explanation for this. They say certain individuals have been born with a predisposition to have this condition. Others say certain viruses or germs may interact with the white cells and cause them to forget their proper function, thus causing them to attack the joints instead of playing a protective role. Whatever the case, it is critical that once this problem is detected it is dealt with before it germinates into this problem you now face, Mary. Waiting until it is so advanced can prove costly.

Facts About Rheumatoid Arthritis

One of the questions Mary asked me when she visited my office was, "Doctor Oyoo, am I the only one this disease has ever afflicted or are there others?"

I said, "Did you pass some people in the lobby?"

Mary said yes.

"You are not alone," I said.

For Mary's sake—and for the sake of the many others who fear they may be experiencing a unique problem, let me present pertinent facts that should put their minds at ease.

- There are 200 different types of arthritis.
- 70% of people with rheumatoid arthritis have signs of permanent joint damage within the first two years of disease onset.

- Although the joints are primarily affected by rheumatoid arthritis, there may also be non-joint complications, ranging from fatigue and fever to an increase in cardiovascular disease and bone degeneration.
- Rheumatoid arthritis occurs between the ages of 30 and 50 and affects three times as many women as it affects men.
- Within ten years after onset, less than 50% of patients cannot continue to work or function normally on a daily basis due to the debilitating and deforming effects of rheumatoid arthritis.
- The average life expectancy of a patient with rheumatoid arthritis is shortened by 3-7 years, and patients with severe rheumatoid arthritis may die 10-15 years earlier than their expected expiry date.

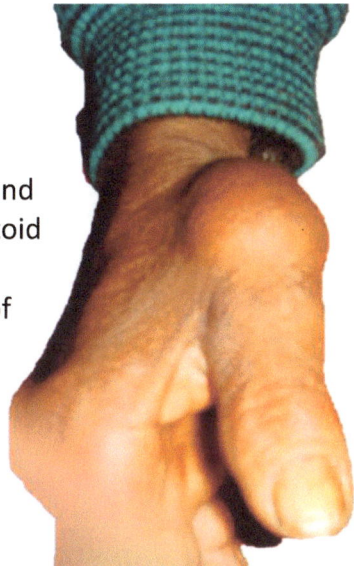

RHEUMATOID DEFORMITY OF THE THUMB

If Mary was here I would have asked her whether those facts make her feel any more at ease than before she knew them. I know she would say they amount to nothing more than cold comfort because they are predictive and cold.

Maybe what would be better for folks like Mary is to tell them how to judge the onset of rheumatoid arthritis. How does this disease present?

The Symptoms of Rheumatoid Arthritis

Listen, Mary, rheumatoid arthritis may come suddenly and last a short time or it may creep in insidiously and last months or even years. Whatever the onset and course, however, the dominant complaint is:

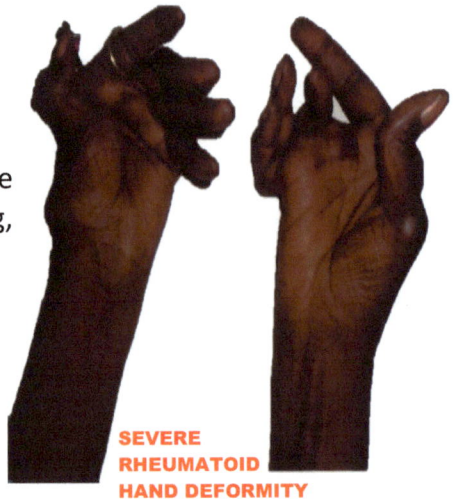

SEVERE RHEUMATOID HAND DEFORMITY

- Pain, which may be described as biting, groaning, aching or gnawing. But pain is pain!
- Discomfort
- Stiffness, especially where the joints appear frozen in the mornings.
- Heat in the affected joint.

There may be times when one experiences "referred pain." This is a situation where one may have arthritis in the hip joint but feel pain in the knee. Whatever the case, we all need to be aware of these presentments so that should we see them we talk to a doctor at once.

Other symptoms to watch may include:

- Loss of weight
- Fever
- Loss of appetite
- Fatigue
- Depression

TRADITIONAL TREATMENT
OF KNEE ARTHRITIS

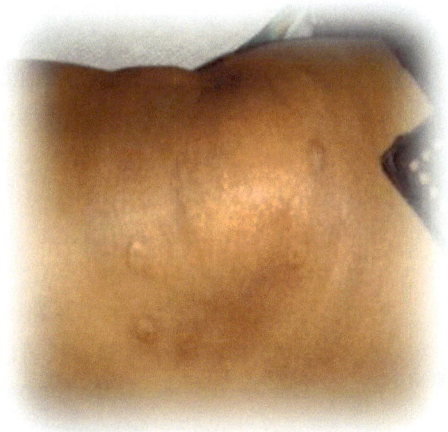

Diagnosis

We discussed diagnosis of arthritis in children and it seemed simple enough. In adults, though, especially if we are dealing with rheumatoid arthritis, a more complicated set of tests is required. In Mary's case I began by requiring blood tests and X-rays. Those were done that same evening. The next day I called her back to carry out a test called Erythrocyte Sedimentation Rate, which reflects joint inflammation. After she was through with this—and hoped I was done—I asked her to undergo just one more. This one was called Anti-CCP antibody test, which helps confirm diagnosis and may show risk of having severe symptoms.

"Oh, wait. I just thought of one more, Mary. I know I had told you we may not require it, but I feel we need to do it. This one is called C-reactive protein. It helps to assess disease activity. If we can do this I'll be a lot more certain of what we are dealing with. Is that okay?"

Mary agreed.

X-RAY OF RHEUMATOID HAND

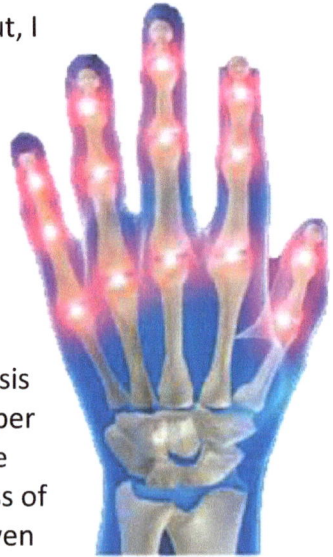

On the basis of the tests we carried out, I later developed an individualized treatment regime for Mary and discouraged her from doing anything outside the range of issues discussed and agreed upon. My reason for being careful was this—it is not advisable for any patient of rheumatoid arthritis to self-medicate as improper diagnosis may lead to improper treatment, possible joint deformity, loss of joint function or even death. Of course I didn't mention death to Mary because it makes no sense to scare a patient who has come under my care looking for help and the assurance of eventual healing.

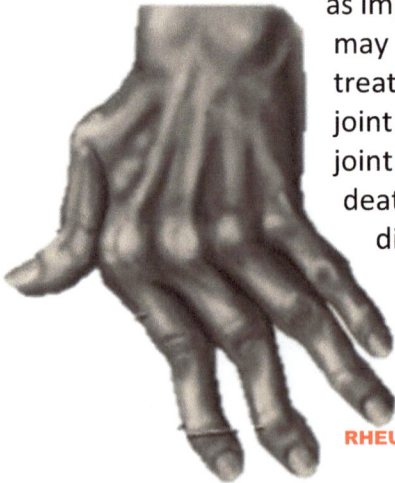

RHEUMATOID HAND

Treatment

Rheumatoid Arthritis must be treated early and aggressively with appropriate medication to prevent joint damage and deformation which may ultimately lead to disability. Effective treatment of this disease today involves hitting hard at it once a proper diagnosis has been made. Such treatment involves treatment with a group of drugs called Disease Modifying Anti-rheumatic Drugs (DMARDs). These drugs are used either alone or in various combinations.

COMBINATION TREATMENT FOR ARTHRITIS

The drugs (DMARDs) may also be used along with low-dose steroids and painkillers. Eventually the steroids may be phased out. A doctor may also decide to inject steroids into painful joints of the knees, shoulders or ankles to relieve pain and inflammation. Because of Mary's intense case, I had to use the DMARDs to treat her. For the record, we didn't eliminate the recurring pain, but we managed to reduce it so substantially that Mary resumed what would pass for normal life under her condition.

Chapter Three

Reactive Arthritis

Reactive arthritis is also known as sero-negative arthritis. It is one of the more common forms of arthritis. As well as the joints, it can affect tendons and their tissues.

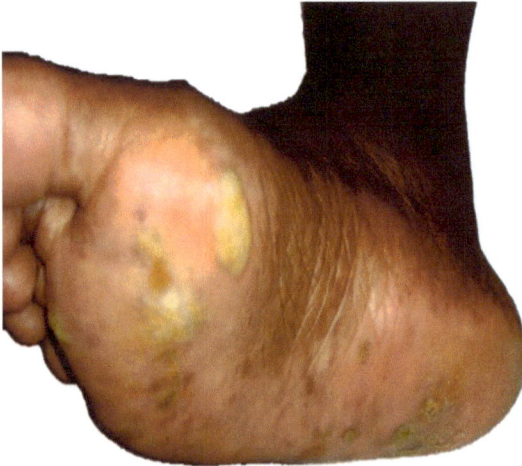

FOOT LESIONS IN REACTIVE ARTHRITIS

It affects young adults, in particular, but can affect children and even older people. It is one disease but it may go under different names like Reiter's syndrome or Reiter's disease. It is a very different form of arthritis and quite distinct from rheumatoid arthritis and even osteoarthritis. It is one of the groups of illnesses often referred to as spondyloarthritis.

The first time I came into contact with a victim of this disease, I was amazed by its similarity and intertwinement to other conditions; a fact that made it rather difficult to single it out as a specific disease. The victim was a young man by the unlikely name of Osore. As its name implies, reactive arthritis is a reaction to an infection. Some of the conditions that may generate a reaction are:

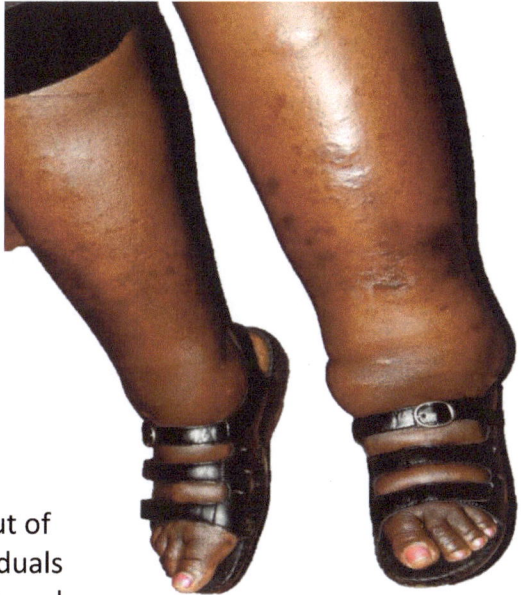
SWOLLEN ANKLE

- Sexually transmitted infection
- Acute infectious diarrhea
- Food poisoning

As many as one or two out of every one hundred individuals with the infections mentioned above may develop an attack of arthritis.

In men, non-gonococcal urethritis can provoke arthritis. In women, on the other hand, cervicitis or inflammation of the cervix of the womb may be a cause. These infections usually produce pain when urine is passed or there may be a discharge from the penis or vagina. The infections can sometimes be very mild and may not even show any symptoms, thus thorough clinical tests, usually carried out by a specialist genito-urinary physician, are necessary to detect or rule out infection. Under normal circumstances, arthritis usually starts a month after development of an infection.

In case the discussion above has been laced with too much scientific mumbo jumbo to make sense, let me pull it down to earth. What we are saying is this—in the event of an infection like chlamydial urethritis in men or a cervical one in women, it may take just a month for a victim to experience the onset of arthritis. In a number of cases the symptoms may be mild and would require a specialist to diagnose. Are we together?

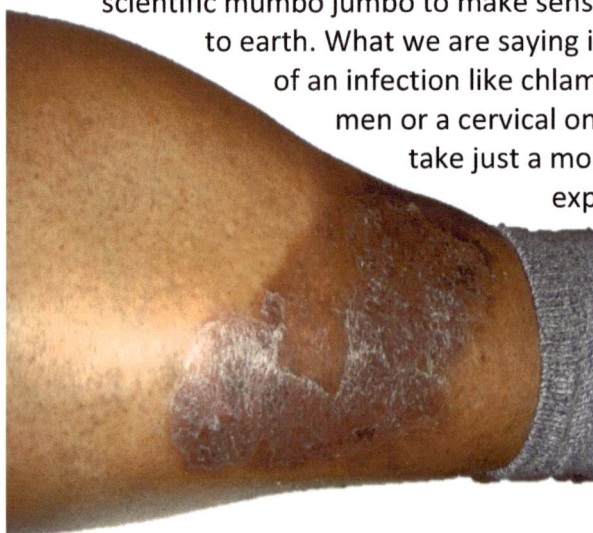

KERATODERMA AS PRESENTS ON THE LEG

Areas Affected By Reactive Arthritis

Osore came to my office rather late one evening. He wanted to be the very last patient I attended to because he felt embarrassed, fearing his illness was more of a sexually transmitted disease than an arthritic one. Only a day before, this young man had been referred to my clinic by a friend who had warned that his symptoms were more consistent with arthritis than a gonorrheal situation and told him to see me at once. When he got to me and described what he felt, I also feared he may have come to the wrong place. It was in that instance that I retreated into my little study and consulted a book I always read when unsure about a situation. In a chapter on arthritis, I came across what the authors called reactive arthritis and the infections that may cause it. Indeed gonorrhea was one of them.

"How long, sir, have you experienced this condition?" I asked Osore when I eventually came out.

"Nearly two months, Doc."

"Do you mean the gonorrhea or the arthritis?" I asked.

Osore seemed dumfounded. "Have you determined that I may be experiencing an arthritic condition?"

"You quite likely are, my friend. So how long with the pain in the lower abdomen?"

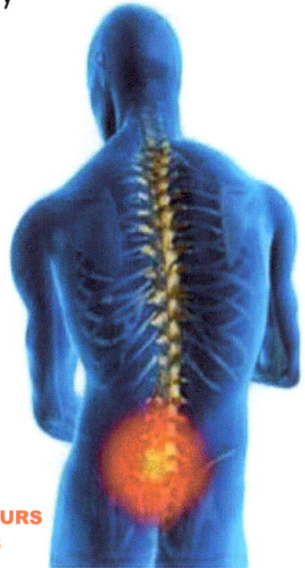

SEVERE BACK PAIN OCCURS IN SPONDYLOARTHRITIS

"Like I said about two months."

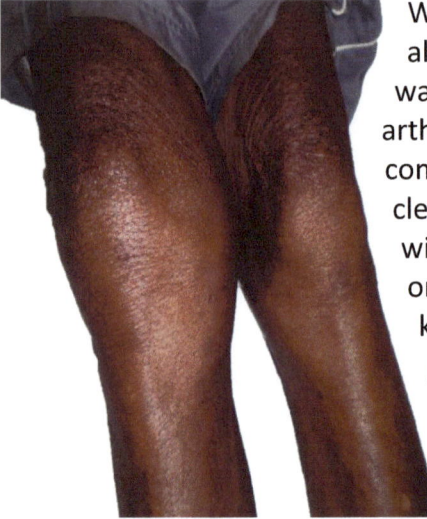

What Osore had experienced all along—after catching gonorrhea—was consistent with reactive arthritis. This form of arthritis usually comes in phases and eventually clears by itself. Typically, it starts with pain, swelling and stiffness of one of the leg joints—often the knee or ball of the foot. Other joints may become similarly affected over the next week or two, with serious inflammation and pain affecting many joints.

SWOLLEN KNEE

I know what I have said above could create the impression that this illness is not only aggressive but fatal as well. Nothing could be farther from the truth. Let me make it clear—usually this form of arthritis is rather moderate and may sometimes affect only one joint. At the beginning of an attack, pain in the lower back often develops. This is usually due to inflammation of the sacroiliac joints at the base of the spine (known as sacroiliitis).

In most sufferers of this disease, the pain is limited to the joints, and in a few instances other tissues also become inflamed. Tendons may end up being affected, especially at the point where they attach to bones. This may cause severe pain, particularly at the heel. In Osore's case, the tendon inflammation was so serious it produced a painful sausage-like swelling.

Now, if you want to know why Osore wanted to be seen among the last of the patients, here it is. It was because of the red scaly areas that occurred around his genitals. He didn't want anybody to hear him explain that to me. The other symptoms, that apparently didn't bother him, were the thick flaky patches that appeared on the soles of the feet. When the skin is so affected it is a condition known as keratoderma and it closely resembles another common condition known as psoriasis.

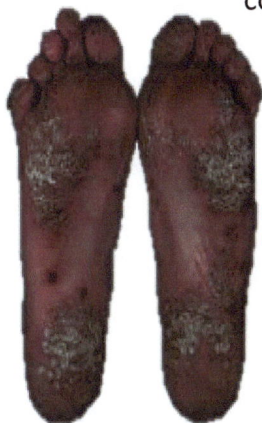

FLAKY PATCHES ON THE FEET IN REACTIVE ARTHRITIS

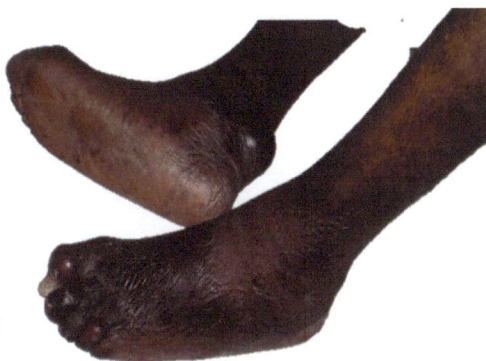

KERATODERMA AS PRESENTS ON THE FEET

The final issue we detected in Osore was inflammation of the eyes, which produced a gritty sensation in one or both eyes. His eyes became red and painful and sticky. What I never told Osore was that the itchiness was as a result of conjunctivitis–a minor condition that gets better by itself and eventually heals altogether.

RED EYE

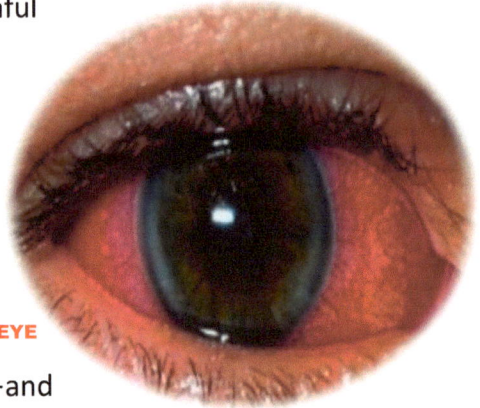

There are a few people—and luckily this wasn't the case with Osore—who the condition may be as a result of iritis (sometimes called acute anterior uveitis), which can quickly damage the eyesight. The common symptoms of this may be grittiness, pain or redness of the eye. Should these be observed, a doctor needs to be reached as soon as possible.

Diagnosis Of Reactive Arthritis

No single test can prove the presence of reactive arthritis; instead diagnosis is made by putting together a number of different pieces of information.

Inflammation of the urethra (urethritis) or cervix (cervicitis) is common in reactive arthritis and so detecting its presence may help the diagnosis. It is thus usually necessary to be examined by a specialist in the genitor-urinary medicine area. Simple, quick tests will reveal whether there is urethritis or cervicitis.

Like was the case with Osore, urethritis or cervicitis may be due to a sexually transmitted infection. I believe I have said enough about this, so I'll leave it at that.

To get to the bottom of Osore's troubles, I had to ask him to provide a stool sample to rule out possible bowel infection. I also had to do blood tests to rule out other possibilities or to assess severity of the condition. In the final analysis, I had to put Osore under an X-ray even though this may not have been necessary.

Look, the point is—by the time Osore came to my clinic, it had been long since the illness had started. When one waits that long, it makes a doctor have to carry out a string of tests that may make the resultant medical bills be higher than would have been the case were quicker action taken. Listen to your body and act when it cries for immediate help. Don't wait!

Treatment

Treatment for reactive arthritis must allow for the fact that it tends to go away naturally, thus potentially toxic drugs should be avoided. Even so, it is important to treat the infection that gave rise to it. That said, take note of the fact that once reactive arthritis starts, it tends to run its natural course regardless of interventions applied.

Whenever diarrhea is the cause, there's usually no need for specific antibiotic treatment. Still, it is important to treat infection of the genital-tract with antibiotics. This should also apply to sexual partners of the infected individual.

Treatment of inflammation of the eyes will largely depend on what type of inflammation this is— conjunctivitis or iritis. Conjunctivitis often settles quickly with antibiotic eye drops or ointment. Iritis, on the other hand, requires steroid drops, sometimes with tablets or injections too.

VISINE EYE DROP

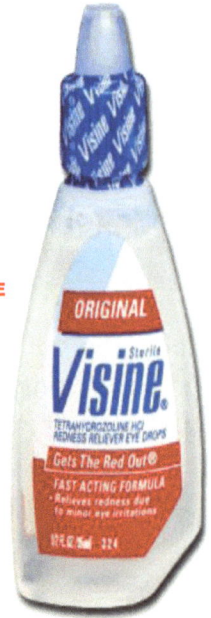

The treatment prescribed for this form of arthritis depends on how severe it is. In the case of Osore I had to use a number of medications to treat the presenting symptoms and end the growing troubles as a result of gonorrhea, but in the milder cases, it is usually better to avoid medication altogether since no treatment will really cure the disease.

Other forms of treatment to consider may include:

1. Rest, which can be achieved by staying in bed or wearing a splint on the affected joint.
2. Wearing pads or well-padded shoes.
3. Anti-inflammatory medication. This can be helpful in controlling joint pains and swelling. Note that such drugs may also produce side-effects and should be taken under medical supervision.

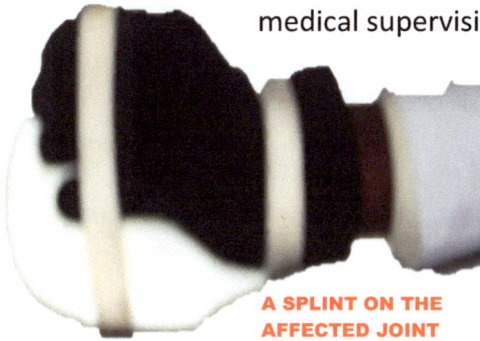

A SPLINT ON THE AFFECTED JOINT

4. Injecting affected area with steroids to reduce pain. This can produce dramatic relief, but such injections should not be given repeatedly.

Recovery

The good news is this—and I confirmed this by working with Osore—most sufferers of reactive arthritis recover completely within six months, although mild joint aches may persist for longer. For some people, symptoms may last longer than a year and permanent joint damage can occur.

Before I conclude this segment, let me warn that reactive arthritis is a condition that can and has recurred in a number of victims, although recurrence tends to be milder and affects only one person in three. It is wise to take precautions to avoid this disease from the get go by using condoms to keep sexually-transmitted diseases at bay and being careful whenever travelling to areas prone to diarrhea by carrying safe water and well cooked food.

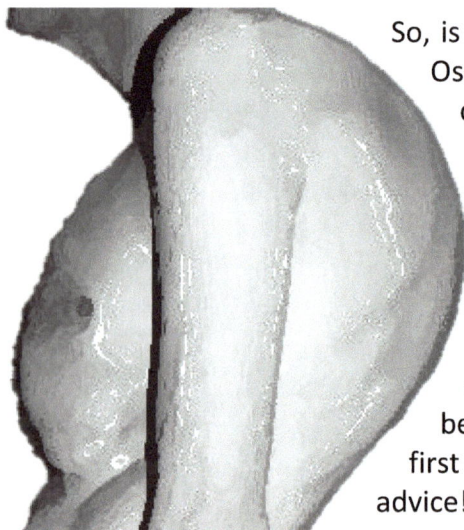

So, is reactive arthritis hereditary as Osore believed when he first came to my office? The straight answer is no. However, it is also known that an inherited factor (the HLA B27 gene) is very important in making individuals prone to this condition. And on that note I end this chapter, but not before repeating this—at the first sign of trouble, seek medical advice!

ANKYLOSING SPONDYLITIS ASSOCIATED WITH THE HLA B27 GENE

Chapter Four

Osteoarthritis

Osteoarthritis is the most common form of arthritis and is prevalent among older people. Sometimes it is called degenerative joint disease or osteoarthrosis. It mostly affects cartilage—the hard slippery tissue that covers the ends of bones where they meet to form a joint. Healthy cartilage allows bones to glide over one another and also absorbs energy from the shock of physical movement. In osteoarthritis, the surface layer of cartilage breaks down and wears away, which allows bones under the cartilage to rub together, causing pain, swelling and loss of motion of the joint. Overtime, the joint may lose its normal shape.

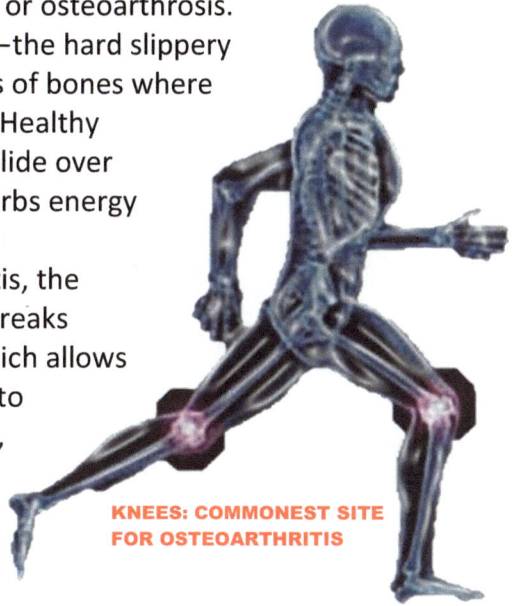

KNEES: COMMONEST SITE FOR OSTEOARTHRITIS

In the case of osteoarthritis, there are two situations that can cause excruciating pain:

> 1. Case where small deposits of bone, called osteophytes or bone spurs, grow on the edges of the joint.

2. A case where bits of bone or cartilage break off and float inside the joint space.

So, Who Has Osteoarthritis?

In the church I attend, there is an old man called John. I won't give you his other name to protect his identity. When John called me one Saturday morning, I thought he was about to ask me to preach or carry out a function at church, but when he let out a controlled sigh and sounded like he dropped on the floor, I instantly sensed this was a medical call to duty, not a spiritual one. I asked John's son to get him to my clinic at once so we could help the old man.

Within thirty minutes, both John and I had made it to the clinic. He said, "*Daktari*—Doctor—this thing is killing me."

"What is it?"

"My joints, Doc. I told you about them last week. Is this a sign that I'm growing too old and need to die or what?"

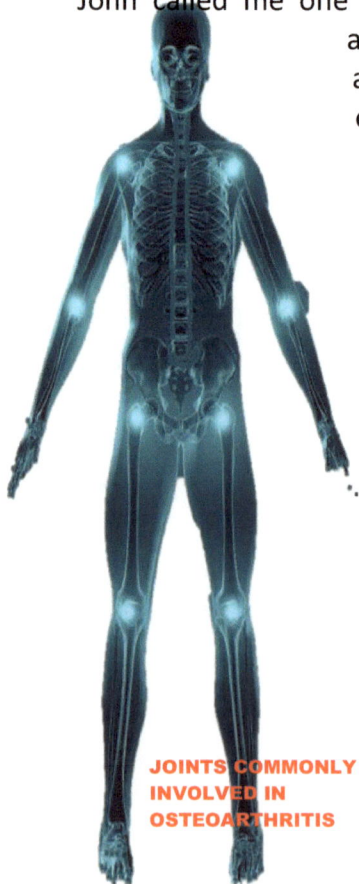

JOINTS COMMONLY INVOLVED IN OSTEOARTHRITIS

I laughed. The old man was one of the most humorous members of our church and I always enjoyed hanging out with him, but he could also be rather stubborn. I recall the many times I'd asked him to visit my clinic but he had declined, saying all I wanted to do was scare him. Now he was here, his eyes deeply sunken in their sockets, his lips bitten in anguish in what appeared to be a case of broken bones or cartilage floating in the joint space.

Before I tell you what I had to do with John, let me tell you who is susceptible to this disease:

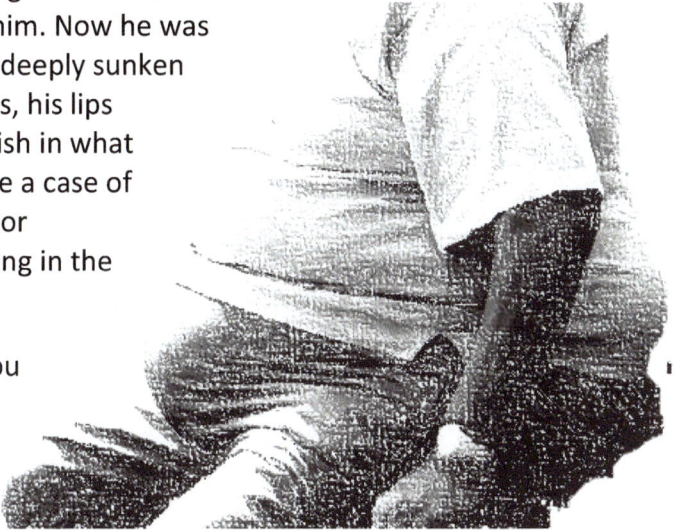

AN OVERWEIGHT MAN

-----People who are overweight.
-----The older folk. In the United States, it is estimated that 27 million people aged above 25 have it. We don't have records of those affected in Kenya, but it's worth noting that as the life expectancy of Kenyans rises, the disease also grows in number of people affected.

----Younger people who have joint injury, joint malformation or a genetic defect in joint cartilage.

----Both men and women have the disease. The amazing thing is this—that before the age of 45 more men than women have it, but after the age of 45 more women than men have it.

----People in jobs that exert stress at the joints.

How Does Osteoarthritis Affect People?

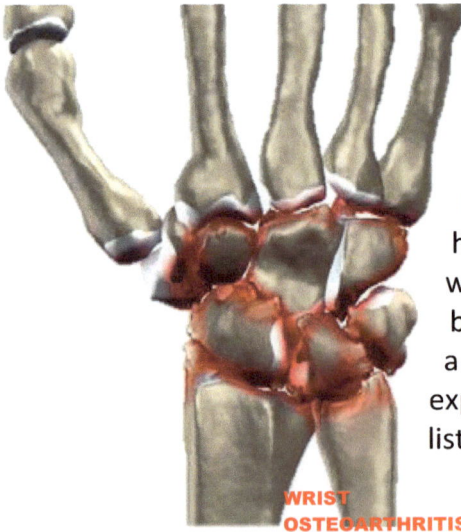

WRIST
OSTEOARTHRITIS

As John sat across from me in the clinic, I couldn't help but wonder about this man. It was like the disease had hit all at once. Hadn't he seen the signs? Felt the gradual creeping? And if he hadn't, did he really believe my warning days ago was a case of bluffing? Once we started talking, a subdued John confessed to have experienced a number of effects. I'll list them here below:

----Joint pain and stiffness, and in John's case the problem was exacerbated by the bones and cartilage that were floating in the joint space. The most commonly affected joints are: fingers, thumbs, neck, lower back, knees and hips.

----For a number of people, osteoarthritis progresses slowly and may not even have an effect in day-to-day life. In John's case, however, the disease had apparently progressed quickly and damaged his joints. As things stood, my good friend was suddenly facing lasting pain and disability.

----Depression.

----Anxiety.

----Feelings of helplessness.

----Limitations on daily activity.

----Job limitations.

----Difficulty participating in everyday personal and family joys and responsibilities.

COMPLICATED KNEE OSTEOARTHRITIS AFTER SURGERY

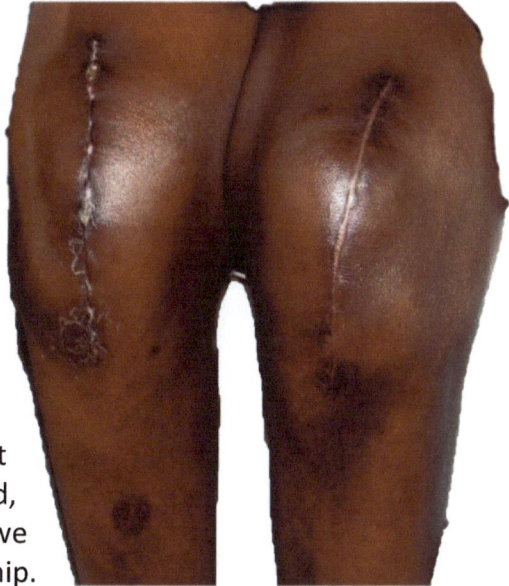

But for John things didn't end there. As we talked, we eventually decided we were going to skip worship. There was a lot to say, especially now that he realized he had to come clean. The devastation this disease had thrown his way hadn't just started; after all, it was something he'd experienced but battled to hide from us—his friends. Now that he was staring the grim reaper in the eye, he even divulged effects of the disease on his wallet and bank account. It had affected:

----His financial base because of the high cost of treatment he was now facing.
----He was going to have to stop working, which would mean wage loss.
----He was going to have to focus on building his retirement home, thereby changing his priorities.

Having talked about all these issues, I looked John in the eye and told him a few truths. No, all was not lost. In fact if he had a good attitude and learnt self-care, he could live a productive life just like others similarly afflicted had managed to do. He needed to start exercising, use pain relief medications and join support programs. Was he willing? It came down to this—either he had to or watch as his life degenerated into a big mess. He could even die!

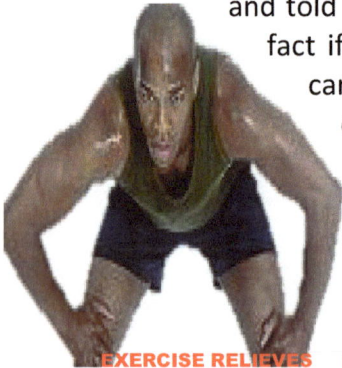

EXERCISE RELIEVES PAIN IN ARTHRITIS

How Does One Tell He / She Has Osteoarthritis?

Usually the disease comes on slowly. Early in the disease, the joints may ache after physical work or exercise, but later the pain may become persistent. In John's case, he experienced stiffness when he woke up or whenever he sat in one position too long.

The joints affected are listed below:

- Hands
- Knees
- Hips
- Spine (either at the neck or lower back)

Let's talk specifics now.

Hand Osteoarthritis

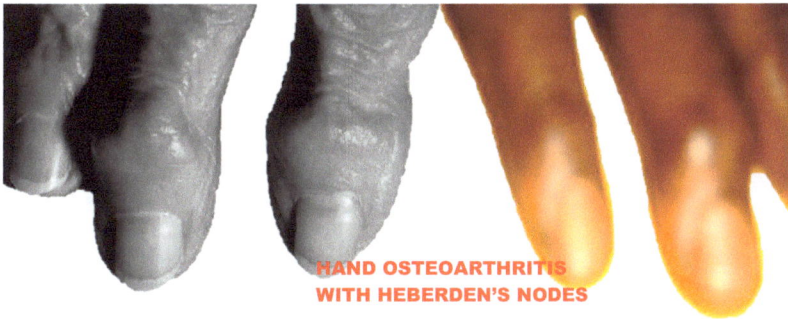

HAND OSTEOARTHRITIS WITH HEBERDEN'S NODES

This form of arthritis seems to have some hereditary characteristics—it runs in the family. If one has it, small bony knobs known as Heberden's nodes may appear at the joints closest to the nails. Similar nodes, known as Bouchard's, may appear on the middle joints or even fingers. The base of the thumb is also a fertile ground for osteoarthritis.

Knee Osteoarthritis

Symptoms of knee osteoarthritis include stiffness, swelling and pain, which make it hard to walk, climb and make it hard to get in or out of chairs and bathtubs. Like in the case of John, osteoarthritis in the knee can cause disability.

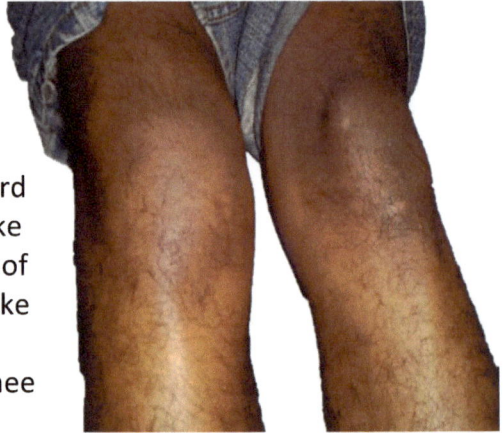

KNEE OSTEOARTHRITIS

Hip Osteoarthritis

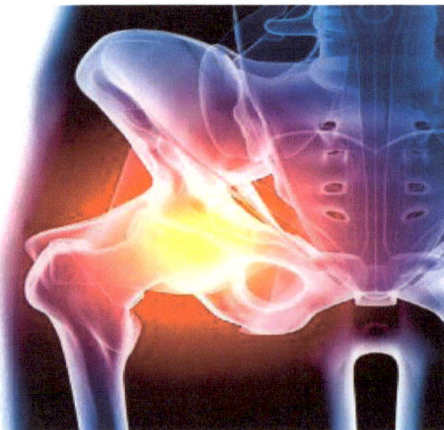

Its symptoms include pain and stiffness of the hip joint itself, but sometimes pain may be felt in the groin, inner thigh, buttocks, or even the knee. It may limit moving and bending, making dressing and putting on shoes a challenge.

HIP OSTEOARTHRITIS

Diagnosis

No single test can diagnose this disease. When John came to my clinic, I had to use a combination of tests to eventually affirm that indeed it was osteoarthritis he was suffering. Those tests included:

- Clinical History: This is where I asked John how, when and what symptoms he had suffered over the past months. I also wanted to know about his family's medical history, whether anyone in the family had suffered this illness or not.
- Physical Examination: I checked John's reflexes and general health, including muscle strength. I looked at his ability to walk, bend and carry out activities of daily living.

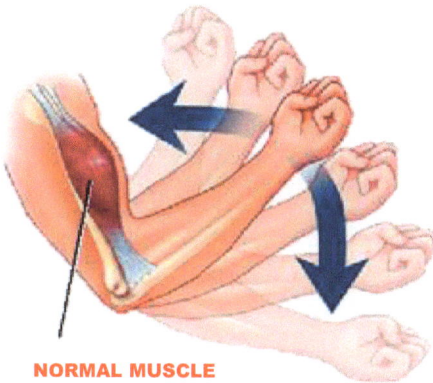

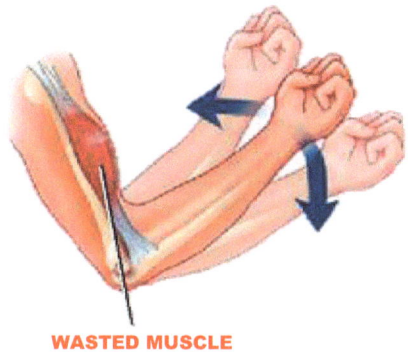

NORMAL MUSCLE   WASTED MUSCLE

- X-ray: I took X-rays to determine how much joint damage we were dealing with.
- Magnetic Resonance Imaging (MRI): John was extremely reluctant to do this test, fearing it would have an impact on his virility. I was amused by his reasoning and had to reassure him that this test had the advantage of providing high-resolution computerized images of internal body tissues. People who have been fed the crap that MRIs may cause cancer need to be disabused of such village notions and let science do what it does best.

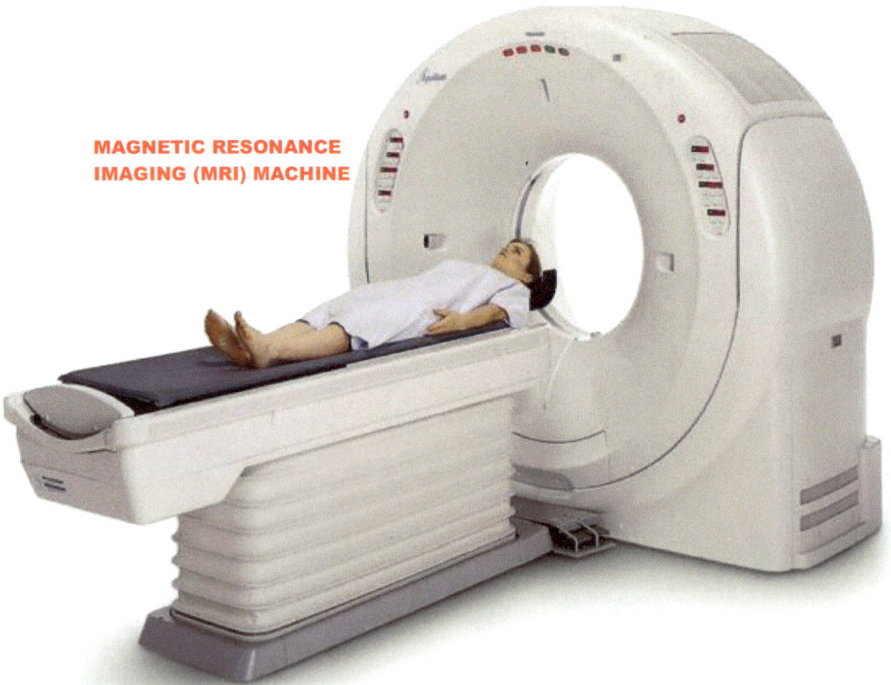

MAGNETIC RESONANCE IMAGING (MRI) MACHINE

There are two tests a doctor may order, which I didn't have to order for John because I was already pretty sure what we were dealing with. For your sake, let me mention them:

- Blood test, to rule out other causes of symptoms.
- Joint aspiration, which is a procedure where liquid is drawn from the joint through a needle and an examination of it performed under a microscope.

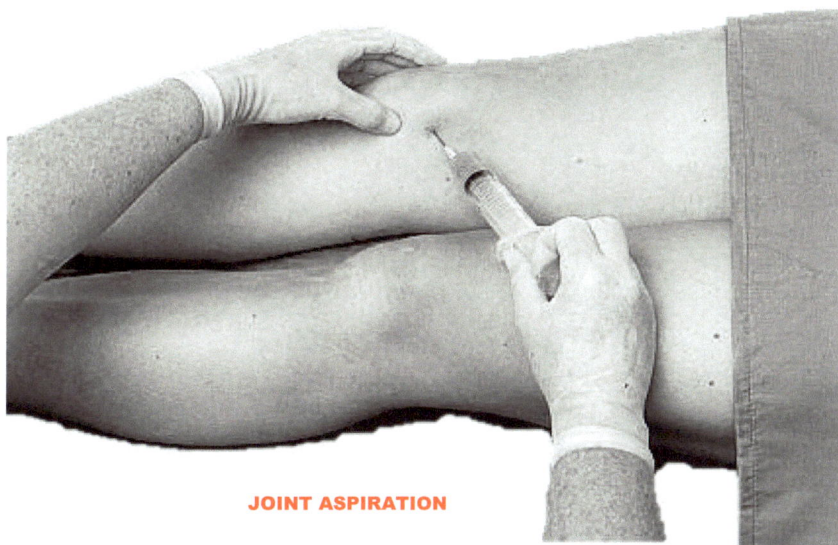

JOINT ASPIRATION

How Is Osteoarthritis Treated?

Let me make a general statement first. Most successful treatment programs for osteoarthritis involve a combination of treatments tailored to the patient's needs, lifestyle and state of health. Most of these programs involve ways to manage pain and improve function. I want us to go through them one by one—at least the key ones. Shall we?

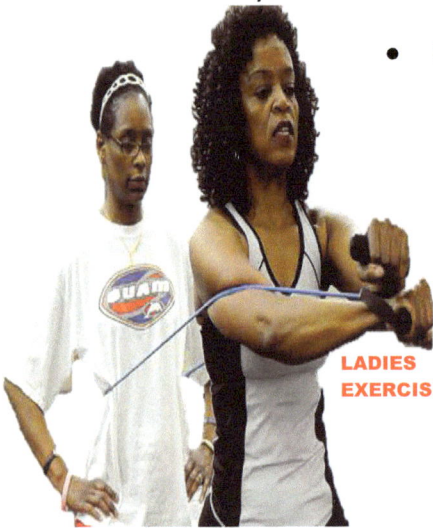
LADIES EXERCISING

- Exercise: Research has shown that exercise is one of the best treatments for osteoarthritis. It can improve mood and outlook, decrease pain, increase flexibility, strengthen the heart and improve blood flow. In John's case, I had to prescribe a certain form of exercise because of the joints affected. Your doctor should ensure that only relevant exercises are prescribed for your specific situation or the whole treatment will be a waste of time.

- Weight Control: A dietician should be called in to help overweight patients lose some of the weight to decrease stress on the weight-bearing joints. A healthy diet and regular exercise helps reduce weight.

- Rest: Treatment plans must include regular rest. A patient needs to learn and listen to the body's signals so he/she knows when to stop and rest. This was the biggest problem with John. He neither knew how to listen to his body nor to slow down when the body demanded so. This stubbornness can exacerbate an already bad situation and make treatment become that much more complicated. Some patients may need to use a walking cane or splints to take off pressure from the joints. As much as this should not present any problems, such measures should be used only for a limited period of time. Whoever needs a splint can talk to a doctor or an occupational therapist about it.

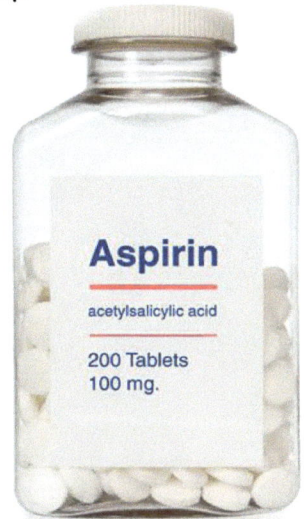

ASPIRIN

- Medications: When doctors want to prescribe medications to deal with pain in an osteoarthritic patient, they consider certain factors: intensity of pain, potential side effects, medical history, and other medications one is currently on. Some of the commonly used drugs are Paracetamol, Aspirin, Ibuprofen, naproxen, and diclofenac sodium. These drugs belong to a group commonly referred to as Non-Steroidal Anti-Inflammatory Drugs (NSAIDs).

There are other forms of treatment for osteoarthritis. Because their application would be largely recommended by a doctor, let me just list them.

- Pain-relieving creams, rubs and sprays: These are products applied directly to the skin over painful joints.
- Tramadol: This is a prescription pain reliever. It carries risks, though, and whoever takes it must be under the constant watch of a doctor.

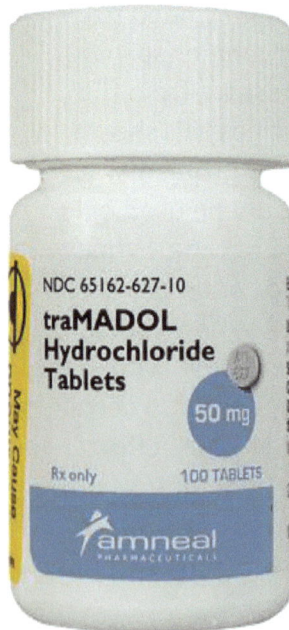

TRAMADOL, USED IN SEVERE PAIN

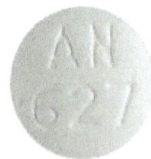

- Mild Narcotic Painkillers: These medications contain narcotic analgesics such as codeine or hydrocodone.
- Corticosteroids: These are powerful anti-inflammatory hormones made naturally in the body or synthetically for use as medicine. They may be injected into the joint to relieve pain.
- Hyaluronic Acid Substitutes: I'll challenge you to ask your doctor about this.

Surgery

BILATERAL KNEE SURGERY
FOR OSTEOARTHRITIS

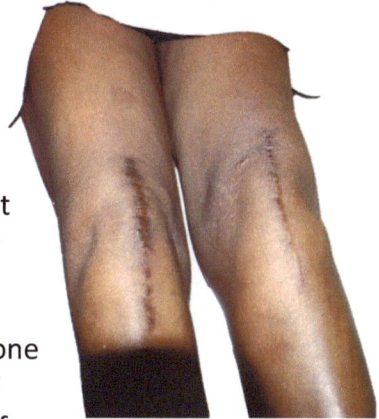

Though this is one of the known treatments, I want to discuss it distinctly. This is because for many people surgery helps relieve the pain and disability of osteoarthritis. It may be performed to achieve one or more of the following:

1. Removal of loose pieces of bone and cartilage from the joint if they are causing symptoms of buckling or locking.
2. Repositioning of bones.
3. Resurfacing (smoothing out) of bones.

You are undoubtedly beginning to wonder why I have dwelt on this form of arthritis longer than the others. The point is—whether we like it or not Kenya is one of Africa's nations where life expectancy has risen significantly and with that comes diseases associated with old age (geriatrics). One of those known diseases is osteoarthritis. In the long run, to save John from himself, we had to recommend surgery. We had to replace his affected knee joints with artificial ones called prostheses. This replacement was a joint made from metal alloys, high density plastics and ceramic material. We projected that, as in other cases, John's artificial joints would last ten to fifteen years.

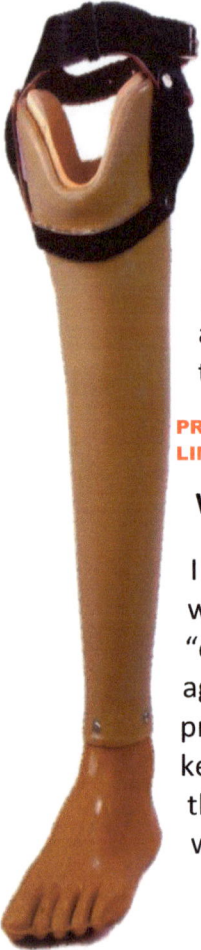

PROSTHETIC LIMB

What You Can Do To Keep Well

I want to end by listing a number of factors that will help you live well with this disease should it "catch you"—as I'm almost certain it will when you age. Although healthcare professionals will prescribe treatments to help you manage it, the key to living well with it is YOU! To live well with this late-life monster, the following six habits are worth committing to:

- Get educated: Learn as much as you can about the disease. In the West (USA and Europe) those affected by this disease can enroll in patient education programs, arthritis self-management programs or arthritis support groups. Here in Kenya and much of Africa, where such programs may not be available, it helps to read books and any available literature. The watchwords are: get educated.

- Stay active: Regular physical activity plays a key role in self-care and wellness. Just remember that it is key to exercise when the pain is least.

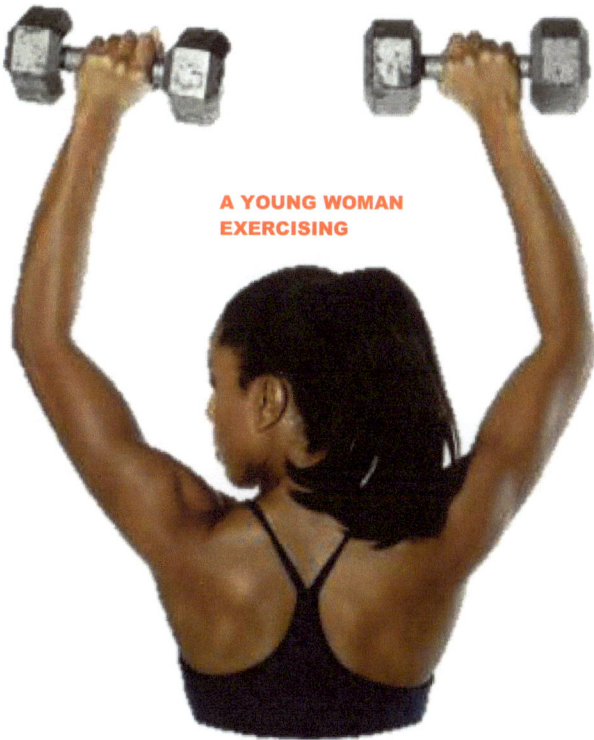

A YOUNG WOMAN EXERCISING

- Eat well: I recall the day I told John he has to eat well. The man pulled his cell phone and dialed his wife. Before I could stop him, he told his wife that Dr. Oyoo says I have to eat chicken, fish and meat every day for the rest of my life. I was amused. The reality is—no specific diet will help contain the pain, still it helps to eat fruits and foods that will enhance weight loss and control. A big body is a recipe for nothing but disaster when one has this disease. Get plenty of sleep. Sleeping well is key to pain reduction. If you can't sleep well because of the pain you experience at night talk to your doctor.

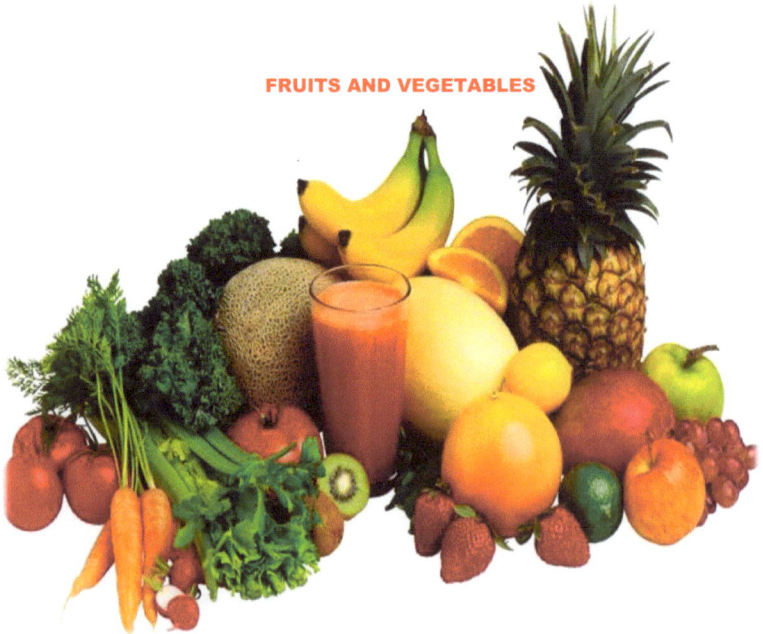

FRUITS AND VEGETABLES

- Have fun: I won't have to say too much about this. The point is—go out and have fun for the sake of being distracted from the pain. If, however, the pain keeps you from forms of fun you used to have, talk to an occupational therapist about new ways to do them. Activities such as sports, hobbies, and volunteer work can distract from your pain and make you a happier, better-rounded person.

- Keep a positive attitude: When I told John he had to keep a positive attitude the rest of his life, he laughed hard, then said, "Now, Dr. Oyoo, you are aware I've always kept a positive attitude, right? Are you saying I have to fake even more of it?"

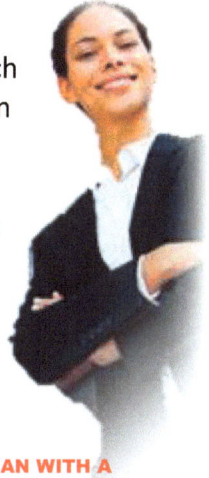

A WOMAN WITH A POSITIVE ATTITUDE

I have said just about everything I could say on this form of arthritis. Like old age, it is surely coming our way at some point, which is why I've taken my time to explain it. There obviously are details I could not include in this brief book because they are beyond the scope of it. The point I must continue to stress is this—never delay in seeking treatment like my good friend John did. It pays to listen to your body and do what it asks you to do, after all, has it not done what you've asked it to do for so many years? The time to return the favor is now!

Chapter Five

Gout

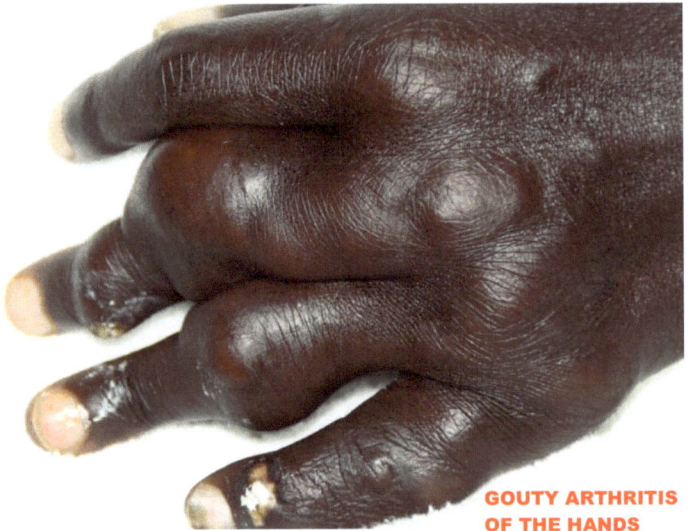

GOUTY ARTHRITIS
OF THE HANDS

It wasn't too long ago that a prominent Kenyan politician died of this condition. For many Kenyans, it was the first time they had ever heard of this illness and even when newspapers described it, it remained to many folks one of those strange illnesses that afflicted the rich and super wealthy in society, not the lowly. Such a fundamental misunderstanding can be dangerous. Let's get down to the basics, shall we?

What Is Gout?

Gout is a painful experience that is common among people who eat too much meat and consume a lot of alcohol. When I told my friend, Sam Okello, that what is killing many Kenyans is the *nyama choma* culture, he turned around and said, "*Daktari*—Doctor—that may be true, but there has to be a way of saying so without offending sensibilities."

Sam is right, but gout is too serious an issue, yet one that is avoidable, so we must take the bull by the horns. This is one of those situations where diplomacy does not help. If the careless men and women I see indulge in this

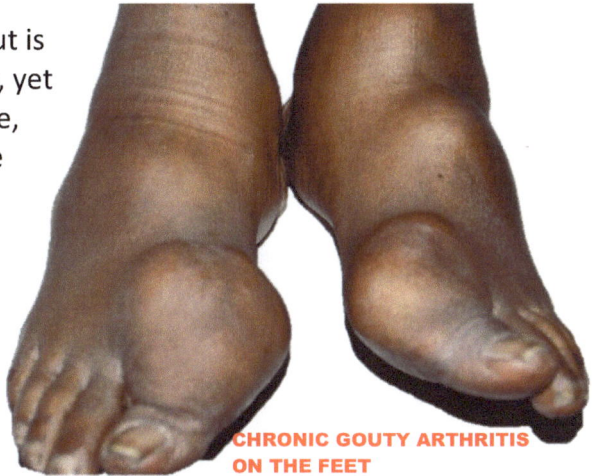

CHRONIC GOUTY ARTHRITIS
ON THE FEET

mess were children I would literally cane them, but since they are adults, I'll limit myself to whacking them with my words, especially when they show up at the clinic crying gout!

So, What Causes Gout?

I wish I could describe this in simpler terms, but I can't. The pain and swelling of gout is caused by uric acid crystals that form in the joint. This is usually from intake of foods with a high concentration of purine. Uric acid is a waste product of purine metabolism. It is dissolved in the blood and excreted through the kidneys into the urine. In people with gout, uric acid levels increase and uric acid crystals are deposited in joints and other tissues. These needle-shaped crystals trigger an immune response that produces intense local inflammation with severe pain, tenderness and swelling, especially of the feet (commonly the big toe).

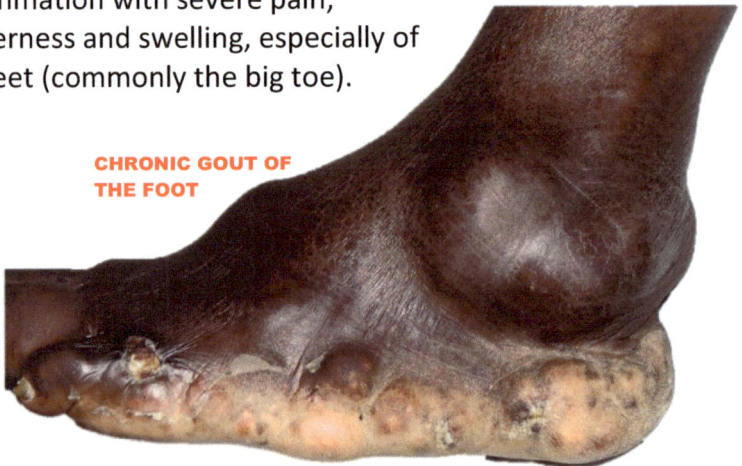

CHRONIC GOUT OF THE FOOT

Increase of serum uric acid over several years lead to a buildup of uric acid crystals in the joint (s) and surrounding tissues. These form deposits that are at times apparent as firm lumps under the skin. These lumps are often found in or near severely affected joints or near the elbow, over the fingers, the ureters and in the bladder. They can cause an increase in blood pressure, thereby putting you at risk of having a kidney problem. This can make life a nightmare.

Kidney stones later form when the uric acid concentration in the urine is too high. This is caused by low water intake, diuretics, and overly acidic urine. In most cases (90%), the victims of this condition are consumers of foods rich in purines, enjoy an enabling lifestyle or are encumbered in metabolic alteration issues due to obesity. Inherited conditions only account for 10% of known causes.

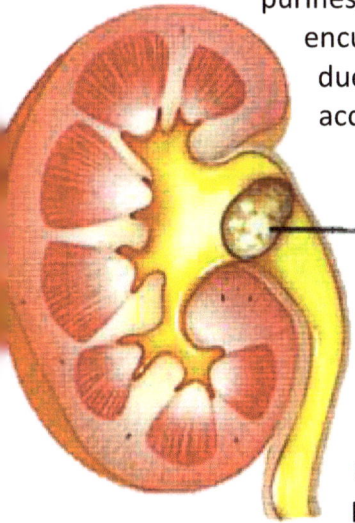

KIDNEY STONE

Dietary Management Of Gout

Because this presentation on gout is meant to be an overview, I'll quickly make mention of the foods and their proper handling.

- Reduce intake of proteins, especially red meat. To be healthy and avoid risks, eat only a plum size of these red meats three times a week. When uric acid levels are determined to have risen significantly, abstain from red meats and reduce intake of white meat.

- Take foods rich in vitamin C. Vitamin C increases urinary excretion of uric acid. Enhanced excretion of uric acid from the body helps lower uric acid levels. Citrus fruits like lemon, lime, orange, tangerines, mangoes and pineapples and lesser citrate fruits like grapes, apples and bananas are very rich in Vitamin C and should be taken regularly.

CITRUS FRUITS

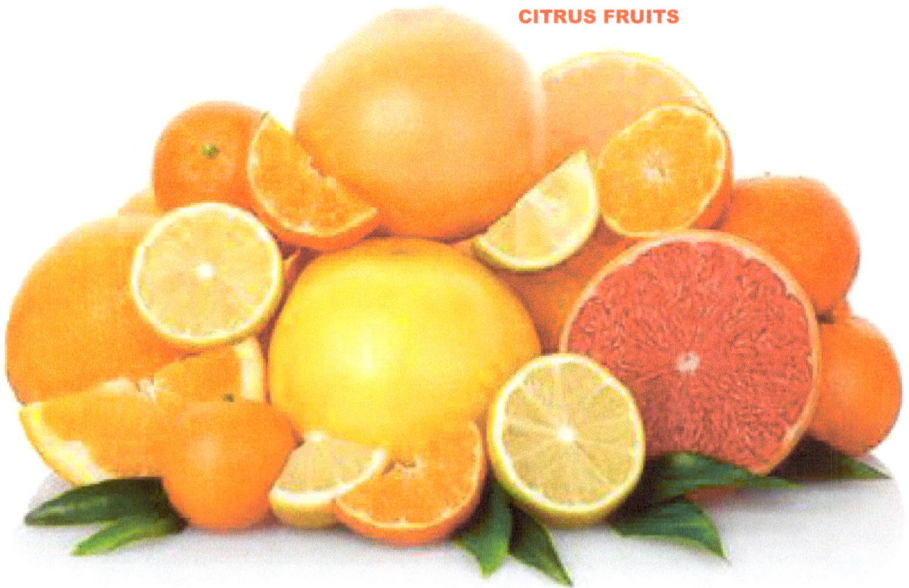

- Reduce intake of Vitamin B Complex. Vitamin B increases enzyme production and leads to build up uric acid. Low intake of this vitamin implies a reduction in the levels of uric acid. Consult your doctor, dietician or physician to ascertain the best form of this complex for you. Avoid over-the-counter supplements.

VITAMIN B-COMPLEX FOOD GROUP

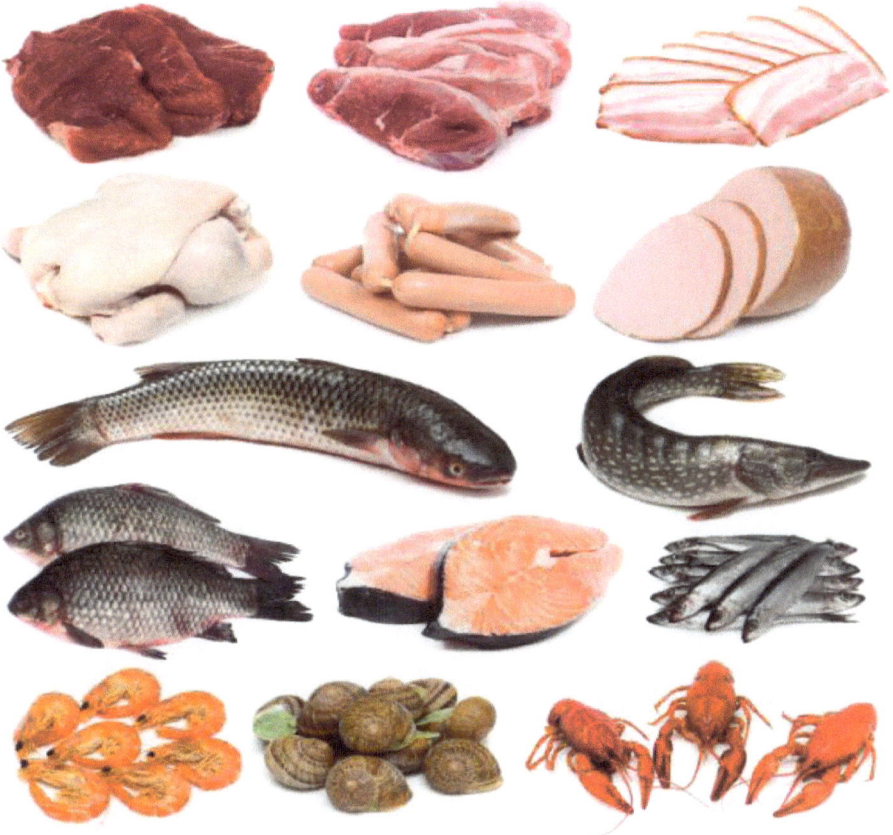

- Drink plenty of non-alcoholic fluids. These include water, fruit juices and tea. For plain water, ensure you take at least 8 glasses per day. Increase of fluid intake dilutes the urine and promotes excretion of uric acid through continuous flashing of the kidneys.

DRINK PLENTY OF WATER, FRUIT JUICES AND TEA

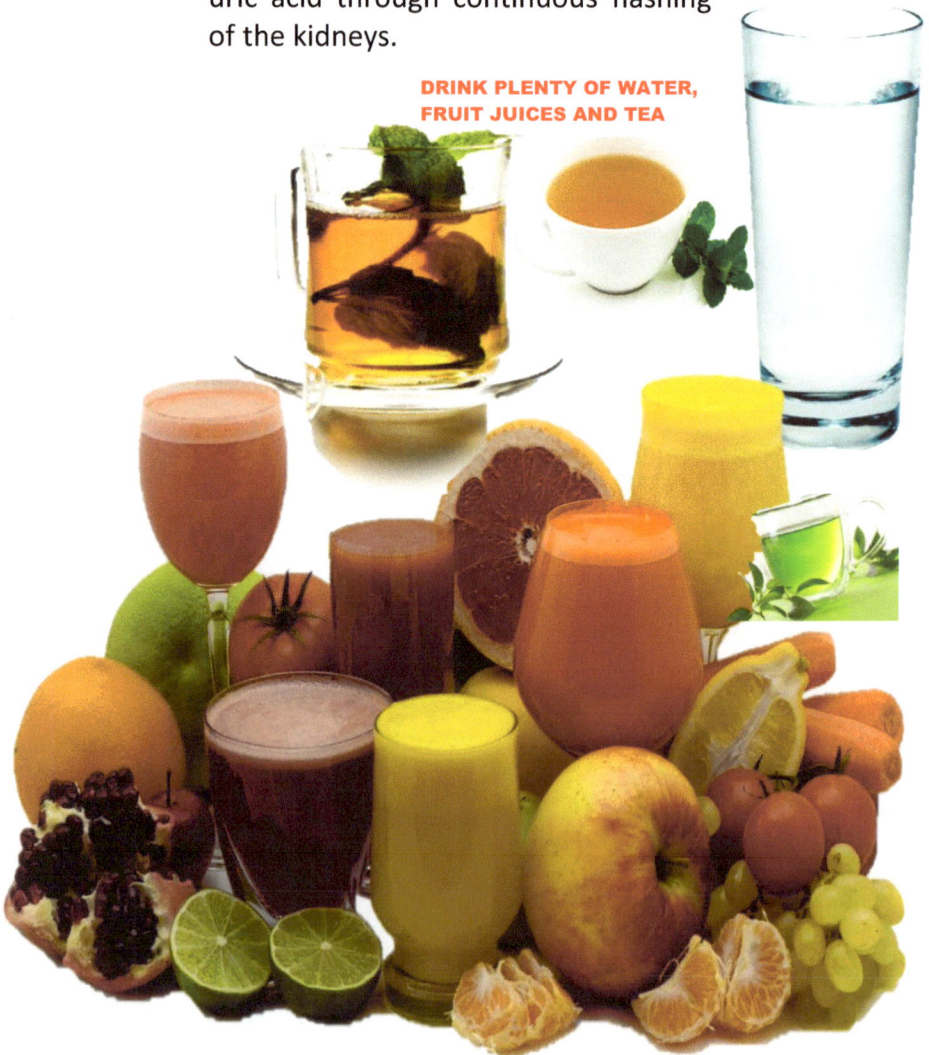

- For hypersensitive patients (those with high blood pressure) and those with a family history of such, have your uric acid levels regularly monitored since high uric acid levels may cause blood pressure to spiral out of control.

BLOOD GLUCOSE AND URIC ACID MONITORING SYSTEM

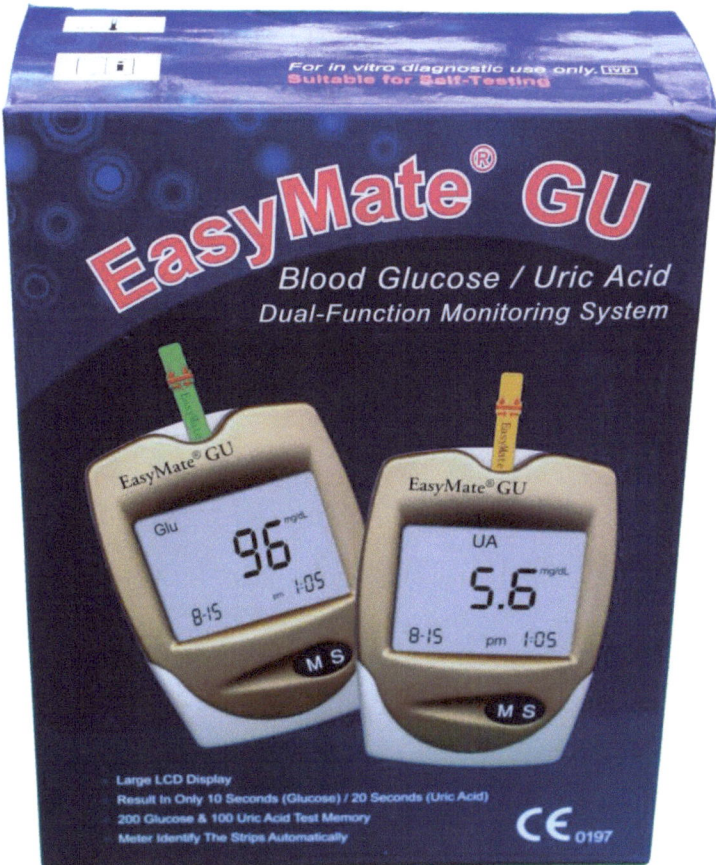

Dietary Guidelines For Gout

I want to give you two sets of guidelines. The first set will apply when one experiences an acute attack of gout. The second will apply at all times. But before we go to the table—where such guidelines are spelt out—let me make this statement. Avoid all foods high in purines as indicated in the table because purines are later broken down into uric acid in the body. Avoid all foods in group 3, limit foods in 2, and eat foods mainly in group 1.

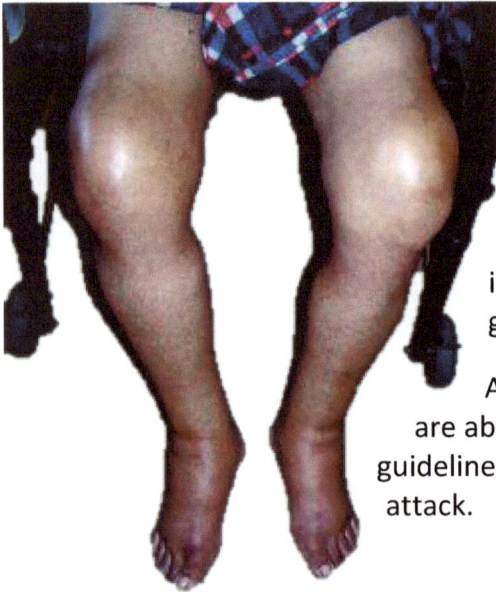

Are we together? What you are about to see in the table are guidelines that apply during an acute attack.

ACUTE GOUT

DIETARY GUIDELINES FOR GOUT

Group 1 (Unrestricted)	Group 2 (60 g meat or ½ cup vegetable 5 times per week)	Group 3 (Avoid)
White bread; crackers	Whole wheat bread, mutton, beef, pork	Anchovies
Cereals and cereal products	Game meat, chicken, goose, duck, turkey	sardines, mussels, roe, herring, mackerel
Cakes, cookies, mealie bread	Fish (except that in group 3), shell fish	Heart, kidney, liver, brains, mincemeat
Noodles, macaroni, rice,	Chicken soup, soup containing meat, asparagus	Meat extracts (e.g. Bovril, marmite, fray gravy, Consommé, broth, bouillon) yeast (including beer)
Popcorn, cheese, eggs, milk	Mushrooms, spinach, dried beans and peas	
Milk products, fruits	Lentils, oatmeal	
Vegetables (except those in group 2 and 3)		
Nuts, olives, herbs, salt, pickles		
Cream, butter margarine, oil		
White sauce, puddings, custard, ice cream		
Sugar, chocolates, carbonate beverages		

The guidelines below apply at all times:

AVOID OILY CHICKEN

- Avoid alcohol.

  - Eat diet high in carbohydrates e.g. bread, cereals, rice and pasta—and low in fat. Reduce fat intake by avoiding fried foods, removing all visible fat from meat before cooking, removing the skin from chicken before cooking, using skim milk and low fat dairy products, not adding oil,

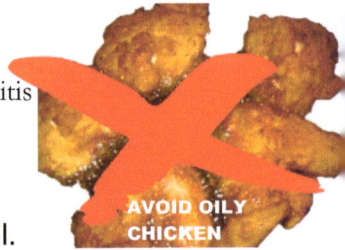

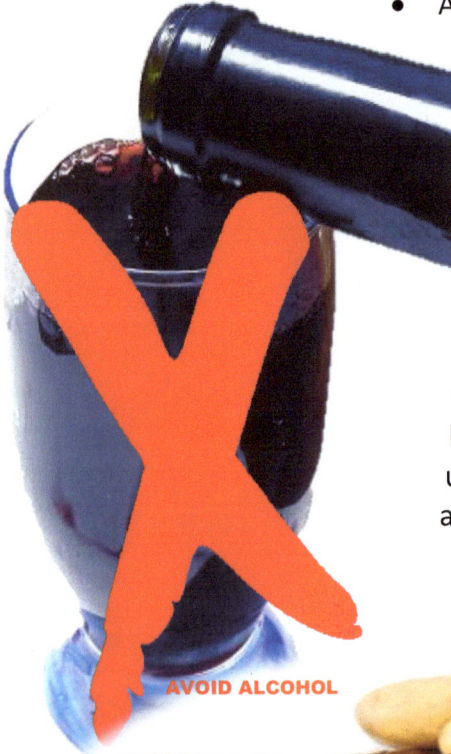

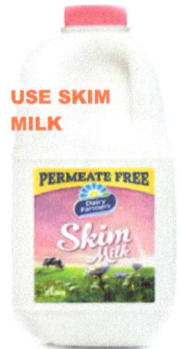

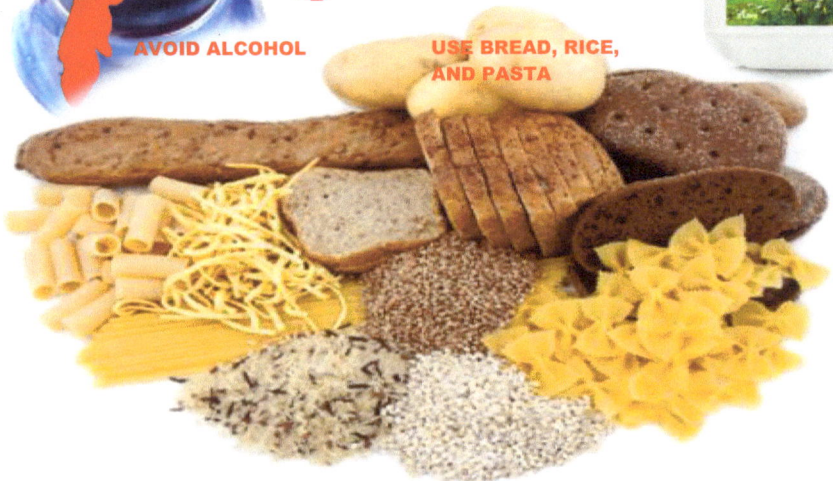

USE SKIM MILK

AVOID ALCOHOL

USE BREAD, RICE, AND PASTA

margarine or mayonnaise to vegetables; spreading margarine thinly on bread.

- Adequate fluid intake (8-10 glasses of water per day) is important, if fluid is not restricted for any other reason.
- Maintain ideal body weight, or lose weight if already overweight.
- Eat regular meals and don't fast.

MAINTAIN IDEAL BODY WEIGHT

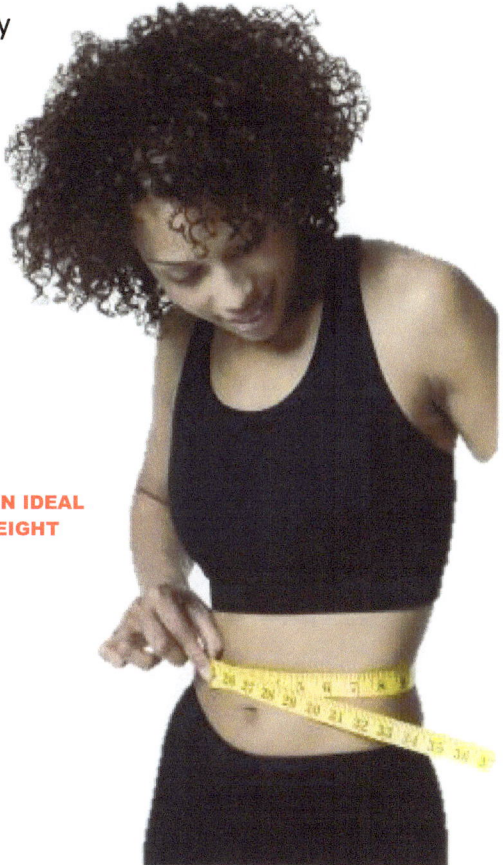

Treatment For Gout

- Pain controlling medication.
- Uric acid lowering medication.
- Looking out for high cholesterol, high blood sugar, high blood pressure and controlling them.

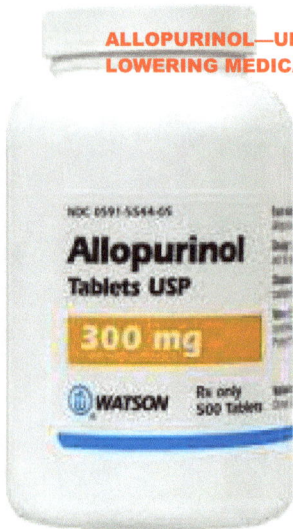

ALLOPURINOL—URIC ACID LOWERING MEDICATION

So much said about gout. Like I have warned several times earlier, if you see any signs of gout creeping see a doctor at once. It does not help to wait when the body warns you that all is not well. Are we together? Then allow me to get to the final issue I want to deal with. This is a form of arthritis that attacks mostly women. It is called Lupus.

ZYLOPRIM (GENERIC) ALLOPURINOL, USED FOR LOWERING URIC ACID

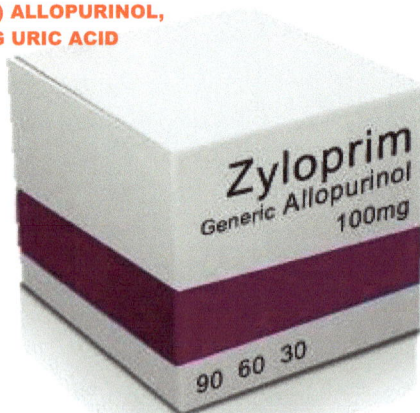

Chapter Six

Lupus
(Systemic Lupus Erythematous)

You will recall that we started this discussion with a form of arthritis that attacks children. There's no better way to wind it down than by a discussion of what I've always thought is one of the most curious arthritis of all. If you want to know why I characterize it as such, just consider that the biggest risk factor for having lupus is being female. Can you believe that? We will discuss why this is the case later.

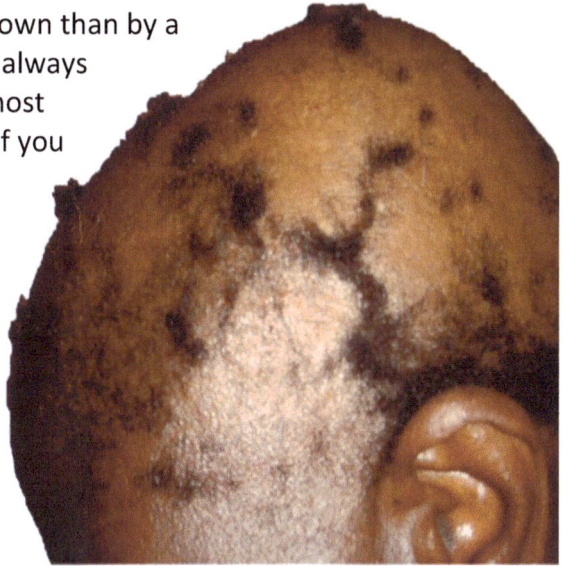

What Is Lupus?

LOSS OF HAIR IN LUPUS

Let me define this disease this way. It is a form of arthritis that attacks the body slowly and strategically, disguising itself as other conditions while targeting virtually every major organ.

Systemic Lupus Erythematous (SLE), or let us just call it lupus to make matters easier, develops slowly over time, with physical signs eventually fitting together like pieces of a puzzle. It usually begins gradually, often with fatigue and low grade fever, both of which could be indicative of a hundred different illnesses. Other symptoms will typically follow, like weight loss or hair loss, perhaps joint pain and rashes across the face. As it progresses, the disease can affect numerous organs. Lupus is a disease—as we already said—that affects nine times more women than it affects men. It occurs when the immune system attacks its own healthy tissue.

Who Gets Lupus?

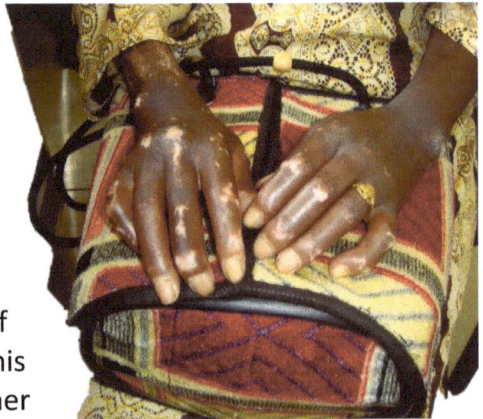

HANDS OF A PATIENT WITH LUPUS

I recall the afternoon at my church when I was called in to discuss a number of health issues. My intention, because the nation was dealing with an acute outbreak of typhoid, was to discuss this topical issue. But no sooner had I started my talk than the audience, made up of women mostly, ambushed me with the lupus question. What the good ladies of my church wanted to know was why the disease attacked mostly women and what the causes were.

It was at this gathering that I made that sweeping statement about lupus being a female disease. With that declaration, some of the men who were in the audience, especially the younger ones peeled off and went to other groups, but the older ones remained with my group. I guess they wanted to understand the disease and help their wives should this ever become a problem in the home.

Let me say this—other than being female, there are other factors that contribute to likelihood. They include:

- Racial or ethnic background: Lupus is most common among Blacks, Native Americans, Chinese, Hispanics and Filipinos.
- Age: Lupus typically occurs during a woman's child-bearing years.

How Does Lupus Present?

This disease presents in different parts of the body. I will take those one by one.

SORE ON THE TONGUE

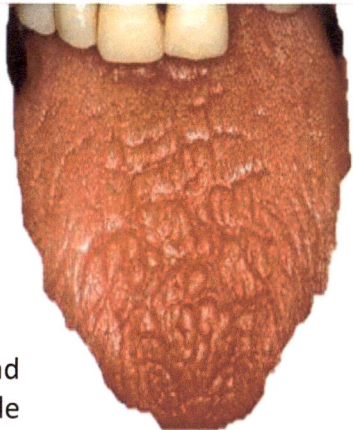

1. Nervous System: Headaches, psychosis, seizures, depression, stroke or other neurological problems.
2. Mouth: Sores on the tongue and inside the mouth. 15% of people

with lupus also have Sjogrens's syndrome—
characterized by eyes and mouth.
3. Extremities: Sensitivity to cold in the fingers;
    Raynaud's phenomenon.
4. Blood: Anemia and blood clotting abnormalities, low
    white blood cells and platelet count.

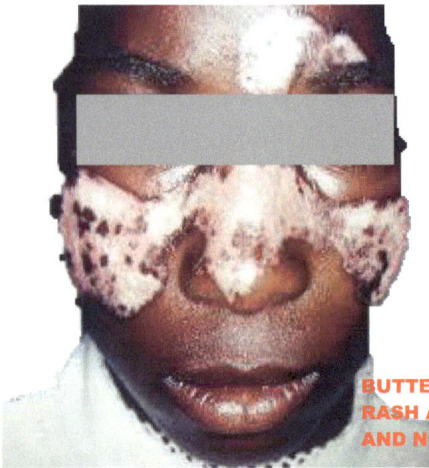

BUTTERFLY SHAPED
RASH ACROSS CHEEKS
AND NOSE

5. Skin and Hair: A butterfly
    shaped rash across the
    cheeks and the bridge of
    the nose; high sensitivity
    to ultraviolet light, rash—
    perhaps even increased
    disease activity, upon
    even minimal sun
    exposure; hair loss.

6. Heart and Lungs:
Inflammation in the lining of the heart and lungs
resulting in chest pain, fever and difficulty breathing.
7. Kidneys: Inflammation of the kidneys (lupus
    Nephritis), potential diminished kidney function.
8. Joints: Pain, swelling and stiffness, specifically in the
    hands, writs and knees, resembling that of
    rheumatoid arthritis.

Diagnosis

A diagnosis of lupus is based on medical history, physical examination and selected laboratory tests. Several medical tests, including the ones listed below, may help confirm a diagnosis and evaluate the extent and severity of the disease:

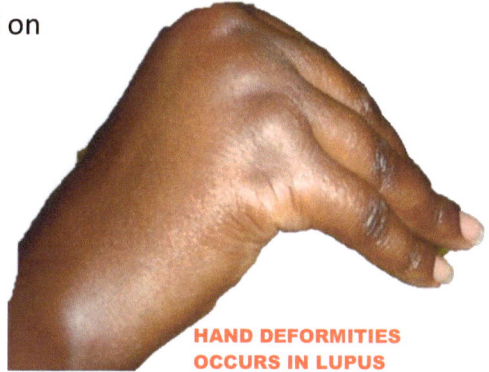

HAND DEFORMITIES OCCURS IN LUPUS

- Blood tests to measure for antinuclear antibodies (ANA), a type of autoantibody common in people with lupus, but also found in 10 to 15 percent of healthy young women. The tests may also detect anemia or thrombocytopenia, a condition that may cause bruising.
- Urinalysis to check for proteins or red blood cells, which may indicate kidney inflammation.
- Chest X-ray or ultrasound to detect heart or lung lining involvement.

How Is Lupus Treated?

The men who were in my group, as if this was the only question they wanted answered, came alive when I got to this point. Could the disease be treated? I didn't want to disappoint them but again facts are facts. I told them that although there is no cure for lupus, proper medical treatment can help most people with the disease live long, active lives. Some of the most common treatments include:

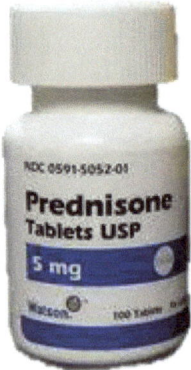

PREDNISONE

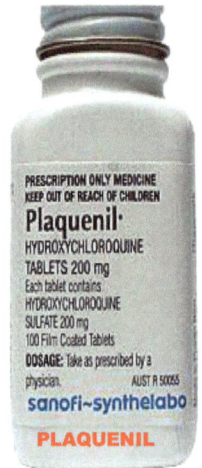

PLAQUENIL

- Prescription and over the counter Non-Steroidal Anti-Inflammatory Drugs (NSAIDs) can help control joint pain and inflammation, reduce fever and help treat inflammation of the lung and heart linings.
- Glucocorticoids such as prednisone effectively reduce inflammation in the joints, kidneys and other organs.
- Antimalarial drugs such as hydroxychloroquine sulfate (Plaquenil) can be useful against joint pain and inflammation, skin lesions, mouth ulcers, sun sensitivity and lung inflammation.

- Immunosuppressive drugs such as azathioprine (Imuran), mycephenolate mefotil (CellCept), and cyclophosphamide (Cytoxan), are often prescribed along with glucocorticoids in more severe cases of lupus, such as lupus nephritis (inflammation of kidneys). These drugs suppress the immune system, which is overactive in people with lupus.
- With research, newer medications are being availed for the treatment of lupus.

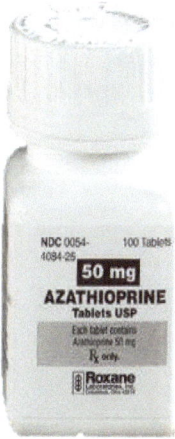

AZATHIOPRINE

CYTOXAN

After my discussion with the church group, they took away the good news that one can live a productive life with this disease even though it can't be treated. Perhaps the one thing other doctors may fault me for saying is this—that many diseases that afflict us in old age are ones that can only be managed and not eliminated altogether. As a doctor, it is my place to tell you that regardless of any condition you may face, you must keep a positive attitude and follow your doctor's orders to a T. And while at it, never

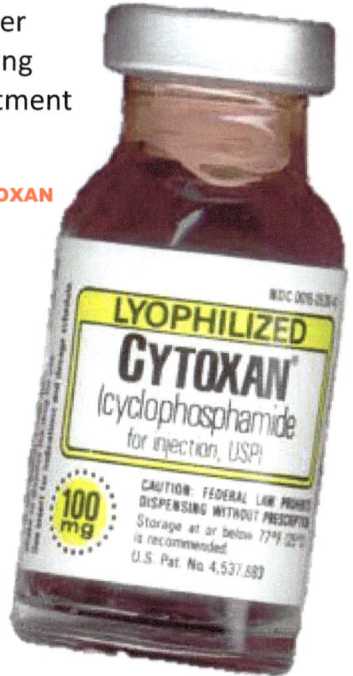

lose sight of the place of prayer and God in your life; after all, He is the Creator of your body and everything in this world. This is the only way to live a long and productive life.

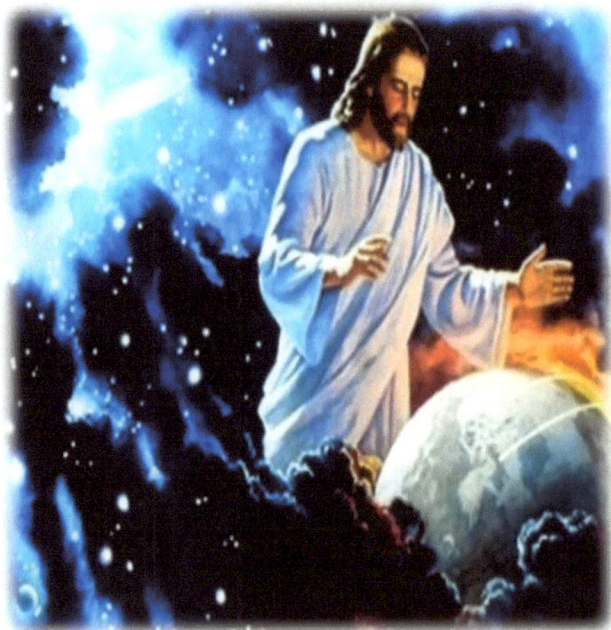

THE CREATOR OF THE WORLD AND YOUR BODY

Chapter Seven

Patient Education

As I promised in chapter one, I want to conclude this book by talking about one of the key issues in the management of arthritis. It is patient education. You will recall that when Mary, Osore and other patients came to my office, they were ignorant about this disease and how to take care of it. To ensure such ignorance is eliminated, an active program of education is required. The first question one may need to answer concerning this is: *what is the goal in the management of arthritis?*

ACTEMRA, FOR MANAGING RHEUMATOID ARTHRITIS

Actemra®
20 mg/ml
Concentrate for
solution for infusion
Tocilizumab
80 mg/4 ml

MABTHERA, FOR TREATMENT OF SEVERE RHEUMATOID ARTHRITIS AND LUPUS

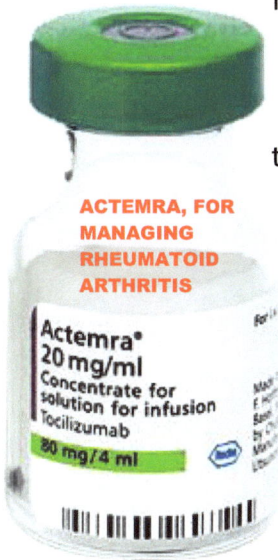

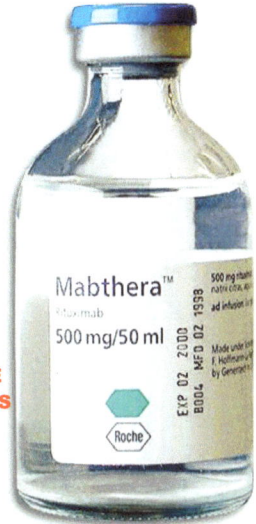

Mabthera™
500 mg/50 ml

The goal is to:

- Control pain
- Suppression of inflammation
- Maintain normal daily activities
- Maximize quality of life

Looking at the list, it may be discouraging to realize—as we already observed—that indeed most forms of arthritis are only to be managed and not cured. The good news is that with education and strict adherence to a doctor's orders any patient may lead a productive and fulfilling life. It is with this goal in mind that I want to propose six factors in the education of a patient. These six factors should form the core of what a diligent doctor discusses with a distressed patient to alleviate the distress and create a sense that the future is not as bleak as it may seem.

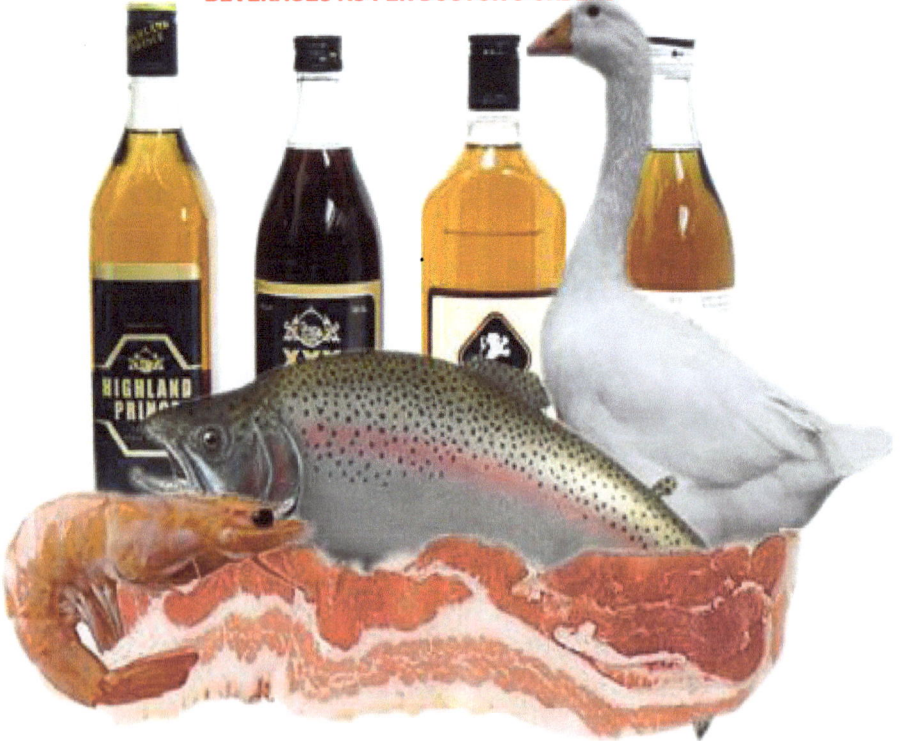

AVOID SOME OF THESE FOODS AND BEVERAGES AS PER DOCTOR'S ORDERS

When the parents of Nina—the little girl in chapter one—visited my office, the apprehension on their faces spoke about the fear in their hearts. They didn't know what to expect from this disease. Was it gonna be cured, managed or would it eventually kill Nina? As I narrated earlier, I treated the little girl, but later had to subject her worried parents to some basics—which constituted their education. Let me discuss with you what I told them:

- Certainty of diagnosis: In the years gone by, it was difficult to diagnose arthritis. Because of ongoing research today we are able to diagnose this illness with certainty. This is a declaration that should make patients—and loved ones—feel good because after diagnosis treatment can be individualized and the patient set on a path to a productive life.

- Chronicity of disorder: Like I said before, certain forms of arthritis can never heal completely. A doctor should be upfront with his/her patient and disclose this information based on the diagnosis.

CHRONIC DISORDER OF THE FINGERS FROM ARTHRITIS

Chronicity should never cause discouragement nor should it be seen as threatening because doctors can today create conditions, through medication, where a patient lives a pain-free life with arthritis.

- Short-term prognosis: A doctor should give his/her patient a prediction of the outcome of treatment, based on the kind of individualized plan mapped out for the patient. Laying out such a prognosis is crucial in building a patient's confidence.

- Benefits and risks of recommended therapies: It is critical to tell the patient the benefits and risks of proposed therapies so that the patient gets into the treatment plan with full knowledge of what's coming.

- Need for ongoing professional evaluation and care: Do you still remember the elder at my church? When I was done treating him that Saturday morning, he looked me in the eye and said, "Dr. Oyoo, I don't want to ever see you again!" I laughed at him because I knew he would be coming back soon. The point I'm making is this—once you start seeing a doctor, don't ever relent. You must keep visiting with your doctor so that your path to a serene life is paved with the right medications and treatment plan. There is no shortcut!

- Family members must be involved: I don't know why we need to stress this fact; it seems to me family members need to use common sense and be there for afflicted relatives, but that is not always the case. Let me say this in as calm a voice as I can— every member of the family has a responsibility to create an environment conducive to the healing of the one suffering this ailment. It saddens me whenever I hear stories of patients who struggle at home alone or with minimal care from members of the family. To family members who act silly I have this to say—quit tripping. Your loved ones look up to you for emotional support and to make available an educational support network.

My Last Words

Friends, I have discussed a number of issues in this book. There are times I've had to be calm and professorial and times I've had to drop my cool and scream. I hope you will forgive this good doctor for any information passed in what you may consider a crude fashion. Take the message of this book kindly and be sure to avail it to anybody you suspect maybe afflicted by arthritis. Help is available!

Mungu awabariki—**God bless!**

Sources

1. Osteoarthritis, a U.S. Department of Health and Human Services journal, in recognition of The National Bone and Joint Decade, 2002 to 2011

2. Arthritis in Children, a pamphlet by Arthritis Foundation, head office Box number 6775, Roggebaai 8012

3. What Is Sero-Negative Arthritis?, a pamphlet by Arthritis Foundation, head office Box number 6775, Roggebaai 8012

4. Gout, Pain and Nutrition, Nairobi Arthritis Clinic, Bishops Road, Nairobi, Kenya

Disclaimer

The information drawn from these pamphlets or journals has been used to form the narrative in the book. Because the book is designed to be reader-friendly to less sophisticated victims of arthritis, the message is sold cheaply to cater to production costs and to stay within the framework of knowledge dissemination rather than for profit venturing.

Sahel Publishing Association
books that speak to your hopes and fears

――――

Other books by Sahel Publishing Association are:

Transform to Transform, by Peter Hamisi Muya
Devil Worship, by Sam Okello
Cartoon Worship, by Clare Kidenda
Remember, by Dr. Vincent Orinda
Arthritis, by Dr. G.O. Oyoo
It took A Broken Arm, by Dr. Harun Lual

www.ingramcontent.com/pod-product-compliance
Lightning Source LLC
Chambersburg PA
CBHW040127270326
41927CB00001B/15